The Skidmore-Roth Outline Series:

FUNDAMENTALS OF NURSING

Patricia Chin, R.N., D.N.Sc.

Assistant Professor
Department of Nursing
California State University, Los Angeles

A SKIDMORE-ROTH PUBLICATION

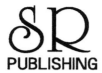
PUBLISHING

Publisher: Linda Skidmore-Roth
Cover design: Angel J. Lopez
Developmental Editor: Ross Odom

Notice: The author and publisher of this volume have taken care to
make certain that all information is correct and compatible with
standards generally accepted at the time of publication. Because the
science of nursing is constantly changing and expanding, new techniques and concepts are continually implemented. Therefore, the
reader is encouraged to stay abreast of new developments in the nursing field and to be aware that policies vary according to the
guidelines of each school or institution.

Chin, Patricia
Fundamentals of Nursing

ISBN 1-56930-029-1
1. Nursing Handbooks, Manuals
2. Medical Handbooks, Manuals

SKIDMORE-ROTH PUBLISHING, INC.
7730 Trade Center Ave.
El Paso, Texas 79912
1(800) 825-3150

Table of Contents

Introduction

PRINCIPLES AND THEIR USE IN NURSING PRACTICE

A. Definition of a principle

1. A principle might be considered:
   a. A proven fact
   b. A group of interrelated facts forming a law
   c. A generally accepted theory
   d. A moral doctrine generally accepted by society.

2. Principles serve as guides for action not prescriptions specifying what must be done.

3. Principles are not the details of a method or a procedure.

4. Principles hold true no matter how or where the action is taken.

B. Principles and their relationship to procedures and policies

1. Principles suggest the action to be taken in a care situation.

2. Procedures and policies are the design and methods specifying the details for carrying out certain care activities.

3. Principles indicate "why" actions are taken while procedures and policies indicate the "how" of actions.

4. Neither written procedures nor policies are sufficient to sustain a lack of awareness of principles.

C. Three principles that guide nursing action

1. Three basic principles in determining nursing care for patients focus on maintaining individuality, maintaining physiological functioning, and protecting the person from illness, disease, and injury.

2. Each of the three principles have been formulated from a variety of sciences and requires knowledge, time, and experience to be fully understood.

3. Principle 1: Maintaining the individuality of the person.
   a. Each person is an individual member of a society.
   b. Each person has rights, privileges, and immunities to be respected.

        c. Race, creed, social, or economic status are not factors in determining an individual's right to care and respect.

        d. Each person has personal fears and needs that are often exaggerated when they experience a threat to their well-being.

4. Principle 2: Maintaining physiological functions in the person. The human body requires the maintenance of certain physiological activities to function effectively.

5. Principle 3: Protecting the person against illness, disease, injury.

        a. Precautionary measures are required to reduce threats to the individual's sense of well-being.

        b. Threats to the individual and to his or her well-being can be physical, chemical, biological, or psychological factors in the person's internal or external environments.

D. Underlying patient rights guiding nursing practice

1. Patients in the health care setting have rights both ethical and legal.

2. Patient rights supported by law are either specifically stated in the laws of a state or jurisdiction or have been consistently supported in court.

3. Patient rights supported by law include:

        a. The right to self-determination and consent

        b. The right to adequate information upon which to make a decision

        c. The right to privacy and confidentiality

        d. The right to safe care

4. Patient rights based on ethical beliefs which constitute high-quality care include:

        a. The right to personal dignity

        b. The right to individualized care

        c. The right to assistance toward independence

        d. The right to complain and obtain changes in care

Unit 1

UNDERSTANDING THE PERSON

In nursing, the person is the recipient of care. The person can be an individual, a family, a group of people, or a community. To be an effective care giver practicing both the art and science of nursing, it is essential to understand the person. This includes an understanding of the physiological and psychological dynamics that govern responses and behaviors to life experiences, changes in health states, and interactions with health care systems. This unit presents relevant, fundamental information about the person and is drawn from both the natural and social sciences. Also presented are discussions of self-concept, culture, ethnicity, spirituality, and values from the perspective of the nursing domain.

SECTION 1: The Individual, Family, Group, and Community

A. The individual

1. Traditionally, the individual has been the focus of nursing care.
2. Individuals do not exist in isolation; they influence, and are influenced by, other people.
3. Each individual is unique, separate from others, and capable of establishing bonds with others.
4. A healthy self, as perceived in Western culture:
   a. Possesses a sense of wholeness or personal integration
   b. Strives to maintain autonomy
   c. Is energetic and directed toward self-actualization
   d. Engages in introspection
   e. Is aware of the passage of time
   f. Has elements of both consistency (sameness) and change
   g. Is composed of a "public self" and a "private self".
5. Understanding the characteristics of the self assists in assessing patient needs and providing effective nursing care.

B. Needs of the individual

1. Maslow's hierarchy of needs provides a perspective for viewing the individual and is a framework for organizing patient care.
2. This perspective proposes that the individual has five categories of needs:
   a. Physiological needs
   b. Safety needs
   c. Love and affection needs
   d. Esteem needs
   e. Self-actualization needs
3. Some of these needs can be met by the person, independently.
4. Other needs are met through interaction with others.
5. Some needs may require nursing intervention in order to be satisfactorily met.
6. This model also suggests that a person's needs are:
   a. Prioritized along a hierarchy

      b. Interrelated
      c. Often met simultaneously
        (see unit 3)

C. The family

1. The family, as the basic unit of human society, plays the primary role in the organization of social relations.

2. The family has a strong impact on the lives of each of its members.

3. Family members influence health in numerous ways:
   a. The family influences each member's health beliefs, practices, and status.
   b. The family shapes each member's values regarding health.
   c. The family influences how each member perceives health and health problems.
   d. The family teaches its members coping strategies and problem-solving approaches.

4. There is general consensus that the family provides the following needs for its members:
   a. Sexual reproduction
   b. Economic resources
   c. Nurturing
   d. Educating
   e. Caring
   f. Status
   g. Political and philosophical positions

5. Characteristics generally considered "family ties" include:
   a. Commitment
   b. Support
   c. Fidelity
   d. Responsibility

6. Two popular conceptual frameworks for organizing family information are 1) a developmental framework and 2) the systems framework.
   a. The developmental framework
      - Is based on a life span continuum demonstrated through developmental stages and developmental tasks:
        1. Pre-expansion; the early marriage period
        2. Expansion; the childbearing and rearing period
        3. Dispersion; children leaving home
        4. Replacement; the later years without children

- The theory focuses on developmental tasks and role expectations of parents and children throughout the life cycle.
- The theory proposes that a family's behavior is consistent with its developmental stage.
- The theory proposes that tasks and the particular state of development that the family is working on are clear and understood by every family member.

b. A systems framework
- System theorists observe the interaction of the parts that make up the whole.
- Basic elements of the theory are:
  1.   Input to the system
  2.   Throughput
  3.   Output from the system
- The theory proposes that the system attempts to regulate itself by the use of feedback loops. When feedback causes the system to move away from homeostasis, it is called positive feedback; to maintain homeostasis, the system provides negative feedback.
- The theory describes the family as an open system.
- Systems theory concepts that are important for the nurse when viewing families from this perspective include:
  1.   Wholeness
  2.   Circular interaction
  3.   Lack of an identified patient
  4.   Holistic thinking

7.   Family structure, functioning, and form can influence the family's health and its ability to cope with health related problems.
   a. Current family forms include:
   - Nuclear family
   - Extended family
   - Single parent family
   - Blended family
   - Communal family
   - Cohabited family

   b. Family structure involves the membership of the family and the organization and patterning of relationships among family members.
   - Who are the family members?
   - Who performs which task for the family?
   - Who is the decision-maker?
   - How is power distributed among family members?

    c. Family functioning involves the processes which the family uses to achieve its goals.

    d. Factors that can affect family functioning and relationships among members include:
- Culture
- Economics
- Life-style
- Life experiences
- Stress
- Illness

8. Family assessment.

    a. Specific assessment of the family will be directed by the framework used by the nurse to understand the family.

    b. The family can be viewed as a strength or limitation in the patient's environment, or the family unit can be identified as the "patient".

    c. At a beginning level, basic assessment can be performed using observation, comparison, and interview, depending on the chosen framework.

    d. Basic areas of family assessment might include:
- Developmental stage
- Wholeness
- Communication
- Support

    e. Common signs of altered family function include:
- Social isolation of family members
- Separation or divorce
- Signs of physical and psychological abuse or neglect in any member
- Problems with educational endeavors
- Scapegoating of one person by other family members
- Emotional problems in children.

    f. The general focus of nursing interventions for interacting and intervening with altered family and social relationships are:
- Promotion of family functioning
- Reinforcement of family strengths
- Identification of support and outside resources
- Anticipatory guidance
- Improving communication patterns
- Developing coping mechanisms
- Promoting family growth and development.

D. Groups

1. A group is composed of two or more individuals who share common characteristics and meet regularly to achieve common goals.

2. A crucial element for any group is active interdependency among group members.

3. All groups will develop a "group culture", or a set of common characteristics and norms.

4. Groups are classified as primary or secondary groups.
   a. A primary group is an informal structure which occurs naturally with its membership being spontaneously chosen.
      Examples of primary groups are:
      • Families
      • Close social networks or friends
      • Neighborhood play groups
      • Mobs

   b. A secondary group has a formal structure and is specifically created to accomplish identified goals.
      Examples of secondary groups are:
      • Therapy groups
      • Educational groups
      • Task or work groups
      • Self-help groups
      • Community support groups

5. Group dynamics refers to the conscious or unconscious forces operating within a group which either facilitate or hinder the group's progression toward meeting its goals.

6. Group process refers to the progressive phases of group development.

7. Effective groups depend upon:
   a. Clearly established goals
   b. Established group norms
   c. Balanced role functions and responsibilities
   d. Group cohesion
   e. Flexible leadership

8. Task roles that assist the group in accomplishing its goals include:
   a. The initiator – presents new ideas
   b. The information seeker – seeks clarification
   c. The information giver – provides information
   d. The opinion giver – expresses beliefs

     e. The orienter – keeps the group focused on its tasks

     f. The recorder – records the group's progress

     g. The energizer – powers the group

     f. The consensus seeker – seeks to establish agreement among group members

9. Maintenance role functions which assist group-building include:

     a. The encourager – supports contributions to group goals

     b. The harmonizer – tries to reduce conflicts among members

     c. The compromiser – acknowledges and incorporates contributions of other group members

     d. The tension reliever – reduces group tension

     e. The standard setter – enforces group norms

     f. The gatekeeper – maintains channels of communication

     g. The group observer – comments on group climate

     h. The follower – goes along with the group majority

10. Roles that serve as barriers to group process include:

     a. The blocker – takes a negative position without offering alternative ideas

     b. The aggressor – attacks and denigrates other group members

     c. The recognition seeker – calls attention to personal needs

     d. The clown – distracts group members from tasks

     e. The dominator – monopolizes group time

11. Group decisions are made by a process of:

     a. Default

     b. Authority rule

     c. Consensus

     d. Unanimous decision

     e. Majority rule

     f. Majority pressure

E. The Community

1. Patients are individuals existing within a family and within the context of a community.

2. Nursing care must encourage interaction of patients with family members, groups, communities, and various institutions to which patients belong.

3. A focus of nursing care and planning is directed toward identifying and using available resources within the community.

    4.   Definitions of community, and types of communities, derive from more advanced concepts of community.

       a. Definitions of community consider three general types:
- Emotional
- Structural
- Functional

       b. Definitions based on community function include:
- Use of space
- Means of livelihood
- Production, distribution, and consumption of goods
- Protection of members
- Education
- Participation
- Linkage with other communities

    5.   Types of communities include:

       a. Space (e.g., neighborhood)

       b. People (e.g., friends in tavern store)

       c. Values (e.g., religious sect)

       d. Interaction (e.g., cancer support group)

       e. Power (e.g., city council)

       f. Social system (e.g., interaction between family, grocery store, church, etc)

       g. Emotional security (e.g., place of birth)

    6.   Community assessment.

       a. Because of limited health resources an attempt is made to provide services to those most in need. Health departments set objectives and target populations to achieve the most efficient use of available resources.

       b. Beginning level community assessment involves identifying community resources and the means by which members can access and obtain those resources.

       c. Organizing, planning, and intervening at a community level are advanced nursing concepts.

SECTION 2: Self-Concept

A. Development of a self-concept

    1.   Self-concept is a complex, conscious and unconscious, representation of feelings, attitudes, and perceptions which the individual holds about his or her own worth, role, and physical being.

2. Self-concept evolves from past experiences, social interactions, and sensations.

3. Self-concept is not the same as the "self".

4. Self-concept is the frame of reference that affects how the person deals with situations, and how he or she relates to others.

5. Self-concept is a combination of both the "real self" and the "ideal self".

6. Self consists of beliefs about the total subjective and objective qualities the person holds about him or her self and includes:
   a. Physical appearance of the individual
   b. Values held by the individual
   c. Ideas the individual holds about him or her self
   d. Knowledge about the individual

7. Self-concept consists of:
   a. The person's subjective image of the self
   b. Perceptions of physical, emotional, and social attributes

8. Self-concepts change slowly over time

9. Factors affecting normal self-concept development include:
   a. Biological make-up
   b. Culture
   c. Values
   d. Beliefs
   e. Coping and stress tolerance
   f. Previous experience
   g. Developmental level

10. Changes in health state and other health factors can also affect the various aspects of the self-concept.

B. Four components of self-concept

1. Body image.
   a. Body image is the person's psychological experience of her or his body and is only partly dependent on the reality of the physical body.
   b. Body image includes attitudes and feelings toward the body which are influenced by cognitive growth and physical development.
   c. Body image is influenced by:
      • Physical changes
      • Physical maturation

- Hormonal changes
- Aging
- Cultural and societal attitudes
- Values

   d. The individual's mental representation of his or her body is slow to adapt to actual physical changes in the body.

   e. Individuals who experience alterations in body image at early stages of development cope and adjust better with the alteration than those who experience alterations later in life.

2. Self-esteem.
   a. Self-esteem is a sense of self-worth and competency, a self-evaluation that is influenced by many internal and external factors.
   b. This self-evaluation is an ongoing mental process that begins early in childhood and continues throughout the life span.
   c. Each Individual has a need to feel competent and worthy of living.
   d. Self-esteem is dependent on a match between the person's self-ideal, which is influenced by societal values, and his or her success with experiences in family relationships, work, and other activities.

3. Roles.
   a. Roles are sets of behaviors used by the person to participate in social groups.
   b. Roles involve expectations or standards of behavior accepted by society.
   c. Role behavior is based upon stable patterns established through the process of socialization that begins shortly after birth.
   d. Roles involve three components:
      - The individual or actor
      - The behavior or action
      - The relationship between the individual and the behavior
   e. Most individuals are required to fulfill more than one ascribed, or prescribed, role at any time.

4. Identity.
   a. Identity is a consistent and persistent sense of self over time.
   b. Identity involves a conscious sense of distinction from other people (individuation).

    c. Identity is a dynamic state that develops throughout life.

    d. Adolescence is a particularly crucial time for identity development.

    e. A sense of identity results in a feeling of self-integration rather than a sense of feeling diffuse. This provides continuity of the person over time.

    f. Sexual identity is a part of one's general self-identity.

    g. Behaving in a manner that conforms to one's self-concept reinforces a sense of identity.

    h. Behaving in a manner that is contradictory to one's self-concept can result in anxiety and apprehension.

C. Factors affecting the components of self-concept

1. A discrepancy between the "real" and the "ideal" self can be a source of intense stress for the individual.

2. Internal and external stressors challenge the equilibrium and adaptive ability of the individual.

3. The speed at which change occurs is a factor in adapting. When change is slow and progressive the individual has an opportunity for anticipatory mourning, and adaptation is concurrent with the change.

4. Societal standards and the responses of significant others affect the significance of a stressor and its impact on self-concept.

5. Body image stressors include:

    a. Changes in appearance (amputation, disfigurement, pregnancy)

    b. Changes in function (renal failure, cardiac disease, colostomy, ileostomy, paralysis)

    c. Changes associated with normal aging

    d. The value associated with loss of function, or change in appearance, influences the significance and perception of stress

    e. The degree of visibility of changes in appearance or function is an important factor in the perception of stress and coping needs of the individual

6. Self-esteem stressors include:

    a. Inability to meet parental and/or authority figure expectations

    b. Harsh unwarranted criticism

    c. Inconsistent punishment

    d. Sibling rivalry

      e. Repeated defeats, or failures, in relationships or work
         endeavors

      f. Illness, injury, or disease which interrupts or changes life
        patterns

7. Role stressors.

      a. Role stressors involve transitions associated with
         maturational and situational experiences and alterations
         in health state.

      b. Role transitions may result in:
- Role conflict
- Role ambiguity
- Role strain

      c. There are four basic types of role conflict:
- Interpersonal conflict, or incompatible expectations among individuals regarding role expectations
- Inter-role conflict, or expectations of one role in opposition to expectations of those of another role
- Person-role conflict, or a violation of one's values
- Role overload, or excessive number of role demands

      d. Role ambiguity involves unclear role expectations and the inability to predict the reaction of others to one's behavior.

      e. Role strain is a feeling of frustration resulting from the individual's feeling inadequate or unsuited to a role.

10. Identity stressors

      a. Identity stressors can be experienced at any time throughout the lifespan.

      b. Identity stressors include:
- Limitations in meeting life goals
- Changes associated with aging
- Challenges to the person's value system
- Social or cultural stressors

      c. Inability to adapt to identity stressors may result in identity confusion and, in extreme cases, depersonalization.

D. Altered self-concept

1. Not all individuals will respond to the same situations with the same degree of stress.

2. The person's perception of stress is an important factor influencing adaptive responses.

3. A person does not have to understand the stressor to feel the stress.

4. Each person has learned patterns of behavior that he or she uses to cope and adapt to stressors.

5. Behaviors associated with an alteration in self-concept include:

    a. Subtle emotional changes that may be blunted, inappropriate, or intense. These include:
- Depersonalization
- Hopelessness
- Helplessness
- Alienation
- Fear of rejection
- Anger
- Sadness
- Shame or guilt
- Worthlessness
- Anxiety
- Depression

    b. Subtle behavioral changes that may be blunted, inappropriate, or intense. These include:
- Lack of interest in activities
- Inability to make decisions
- Social withdrawal
- Avoiding looking at altered body part
- Avoiding discussion of limitations
- Hostility
- Increasing dependence
- Reluctance to ask for assistance
- Suspicion of others
- Self-destructive behaviors

6. Nursing assessment of self-concept should include consideration of actual and potential self-concept stressors and observation of behavior associated with altered self-concept.

E. Assisting the patient to reach long term-goals when experiencing an alteration in self-concept or attaining a more positive self-concept include:

1. Assisting the patient in developing insight and expanding their self-awareness regarding actual or potential stressors

2. Encouraging the patient in self-exploration

3. Assisting the patient in realistic self-evaluation

    4.   Assisting the patient in formulating realistic goals regarding adaptation

    5.   Assisting the patient in achieving realistic goals

    6.   Restoration of a realistic body image

F. Nursing measures for adjusting to an alteration in body image

    1.   Identifying concerns resulting from physical alterations

    2.   Encouraging open discussion of feelings related to the changes

    3.   Demonstrating acceptance of physical body changes

    4.   Encouraging participation in decision-making and problem-solving

    5.   Assisting with meeting physical needs

    6.   Encouraging patient participation in the care of affected body part

    7.   Teaching patient and family to focus on patient's abilities instead of limitations resulting from physical changes

    8.   Referring the patient and family to appropriate self-help groups

SECTION 3: Spirituality

A. Spiritual health

    1.   Spirituality is a component of human nature that nourishes and sustains the essence of life.

    2.   Spiritual health is an awareness of a supreme presence existing with, or existing in, each individual.

    3.   Spiritual distress is a state of disruption in life principles which integrate and transcends ones biological and psychological nature.

    4.   Signs of spiritual distress include:
       a. Guilt
       b. Irascibility
       c. Lack of forgiveness of self and others
       d. Vindictiveness

    5.   Religion is related to the practices, rites, and rituals of organized spiritual groups.

6. Although spiritual care includes religious beliefs and rituals, it is not limited to the practices and dogma of religions.

7. Faith refers to a way of relating to self, others, and a supreme being, with that supreme being as a center.

8. Spirituality develops across the life span, demonstrated through an increasing awareness of the meanings, purposes, and values of life.
    a. Horizontal spiritual development involves establishing meaningful relationships with others, a strong personal identity, and a feeling of positive self-worth.
    b. Vertical spiritual development involves developing relationships with a supreme being.

9. Agnostics believe that the existence of a higher power cannot be known.

10. Atheism is a denial of the existence of a God.

B. Spiritual and religious aspects of health influence

1. All individuals have the need to feel loved, a need for relatedness, and relief from guilt.

2. The spiritual nature of a person assists them in finding meaning in life, suffering, pain, illness, and death.

3. Spirituality aids in sustaining the patient with significant objects, symbols, practices, and rituals to endure times of difficulty or distress.

4. In some belief systems, disease is perceived as part of a divine plan to test the individual's faith and patience.

5. In other belief systems disease, illness, injury, pain, and suffering may be a form of punishment for sins or wrong-doing by the individual.

6. Spirituality and religion influence a patient's:
    a. Beliefs about health
    b. Beliefs about birth
    c. Beliefs about diet
    d. Beliefs about health crisis
    e. Beliefs about death

C. Spiritual health and the nursing process

1. By exploring the patient's symbolic and spiritual supports, providing spiritual resources, suggesting alternative beliefs, or sharing beliefs in a non-judgmental manner, nursing

care can assist patients to find significance in suffering, as well as tolerance, and peace.

2. When assessing the patient's spiritual needs, consideration should be given to:
   a. The patient's idea of a Supreme Being
   b. The patient's sources of strength and hope
   c. The significance to a patient of his or her religious practices and rituals
   d. The patient's perception of the relationship between spiritual beliefs and health
3. The patient's demonstration of contradictory actions or attitudes may be an indicator of spiritual distress.
4. Resources such as family members, clergy, pastoral care department, and other health team members, should be used to help patients maintain or regain their spiritual health.

SECTION 4: Values in the Nursing Context

A. Definition and function of values

1. Values serve a variety of functions for individuals.
   a. They shape the perceptions that individuals have of other people.
   b. They provide a framework for acceptable behavior.
   c. They give meaning to life and provide a reason for selecting certain actions.
   d. They reflect a person's identity.
2. A realistic value system allows a person flexibility in attitudes, behaviors, and feelings, to achieve life satisfaction.
3. Nurses have a set of personal values and a set of professional values which they use in their practice.
4. In the health care setting the values of the nurse, patient, and society, intersect.
5. It is essential that the nurse become aware of his or her personal and professional value sets so that they can most effectively assist patients to become aware of their own values and to see how they are influenced by those values.
6. There are two classifications of values.
   a. Terminal values reflecting desired end states or goals.
   b. Instrumental values reflecting modes of conduct.

7. When clearly identified and affirmed, values increase the patient's ability to make objective decisions about nursing care and health care.

B. **Value formation**
   1. Values are learned through observations and acquired through life experiences.
   2. Value formation begins early in a child's development, although the modification and reinforcement of values continue over the life span.
   3. Values are not learned though a deliberate process, or through conscious selection, but rather through the process of socialization.
   4. Values are transmitted through a variety of mechanisms.
      a. Modeling the values of others
      b. Moralizing from an existing values framework
      c. Experiencing opportunities to make responsible choices
      d. Allowing children to "do their own thing" (Laissez-Faire)
   5. Developmental level significantly influences the way values are formed and expressed.
   6. Value development and modification is subjected to various sociocultural influences, including:
      a. Social settings
      b. Economic background
      c. Spiritual background
      d. Cultural background

C. **Modification of values**
   1. Individual values are modified as the person matures and experiences new situations.
   2. The process of values clarification can help both nurse and patient gain insight into the manner in which personal and professional values influence behavior.
   3. Values clarification involves strategies used to explore the meaning of values and behaviors.
   4. The valuing process includes:
      a. Freely choosing among alternatives after considering all the consequences of each choice.
      b. Prizing, cherishing, and publicly affirming the choice made.

    c. Acting with consistency toward one's beliefs by making the choice part of one's behavior.

5. Values clarification is an important nursing intervention when assessment of the patient's behavior indicates that values may be ambiguous or not clearly directed.

6. Behaviors indicating a patient's need for value clarification include:
   a. Apathy
   b. Flightiness
   c. Inconsistency
   d. Drifting
   e. Over-conforming
   f. Playing the role of the "perfect patient"

D. Professional practice and values

1. Nursing has a code of ethics which directs nursing action.

2. Nurses usually become most aware of the ethical principles and values they possess when they are confronted with ethical dilemmas in practice.

3. An ethical dilemma involves the "ought" and "should" of behavior.

4. Ethical dilemmas in the nursing domain are often the result of technology, specialization of care, and resource limitations.

5. Ethical principles often questioned in the nursing context include:
   a. Fidelity (maintaining loyalty)
   b. Veracity (truth telling)
   c. Autonomy/self-determination (freedom to choose)
   d. Nonmalevolence (desire to do no harm)

SECTION 5: Culture and Ethnicity in the Nursing Context

A. Culture and ethnicity

1. All people share in some culture.

2. Nursing practice occurs in a transcultural context which requires an awareness of, and sensitivity to, the cultural needs and differences of patients.

3. Individuals are influenced by the culture in which they were brought up and in which they currently live.

4. Cultural background involves:
   a. Collective standards of behavior
   b. Shared values
   c. Shared attitudes

5. Cultural background helps the person identify what is considered appropriate behaviors and the expectations of others regarding behavior.

6. To provide individualized nursing care, nurses must incorporate issues of the patient's cultural background into the plan of care.

7. Cultural background strongly influences:
   a. An individual's perceptions and responses to illness, injury, disease, and/or hospitalization
   b. An individual's manner of meeting basic human needs

B. Definitions of culture/ethnicity

1. Definitions of culture.
   a. Culture is the learned ways of acting and thinking transmitted by group members to other group members.
   b. Culture refers to the ready-made and tested solutions to problem-solving, transmitted by the group to other group members.
   c. Culture is the collective pattern shared by members of the group and distinguished from other groups.

2. Definitions of ethnicity
   a. Ethnicity is an alliance among people and is based upon shared linguistic, racial, and cultural background.
   b. Ethnicity is the similarity in cultural background or way of life.

C. Influences of culture on patients

1. Nurses must be aware of how their own values and standards of behavior differ from those of their patient in order to avoid the problems of ethnocentrism, racism, or stereotyping the members of a cultural group.

2. The extent of cultural influence on a person is individualistic.

3. Culture is never acquired as a complete or absolute pattern.

4. Individual differences among members of a cultural group are based upon:
   a. Age
   b. Religion
   c. Language and dialect

    d. Gender identify
    e. Socioeconomic level and background
    f. Geographical location in country of origin
    g. Geographical location of current country of residence
    h. History of the subculture subgroup of the person
    i. Amount and type of contact between youth and elders
    j. Degree of acculturation into the current country of residence

D. Differences and similarities among cultural and ethnic groups

  1. Group cultural characteristics vary greatly with regard to:
    a. Susceptibility to disease
    b. Use of language
    c. Foods and eating habits
    d. Time orientation
    e. Use of personal space and territoriality
    f. Attitudes toward the family
    g. Emotional reactions and expressions
    h. Pain responses and expressions
    i. Mental and emotional health
    j. Health and illness beliefs and practices

E. Cultural/ethnic factors and the nursing process

  1. When assessing a member of a particular minority group, consider the appropriate factors for meeting individual cultural needs and understanding the social and cultural reality of the patient, family, and community.
  2. Cultural factors to consider when assessing cultural and ethnic influences and needs include:
    a. Ethnic origin
    b. Race
    c. Place of birth
    d. Relocation pattern
    e. Habits, customs, values, beliefs
    f. Cultural sanctions and restrictions
    g. Language/communication process
    h. Healing beliefs and practices
    i. Nutritional factors
  3. Sociological factors to consider include:
    a. Economic status
    b. Educational status
    c. Social network

      d   Degree of available family support

      e. Supportive institutions

4.   Psychological factors to consider include:

      a. Self-concept

      b. Mental and behavioral processes and characteristics

      c. Religious influences

      d. Responses to stress and discomfort

5.   Biological/physiological factors to consider include:

      a. Racial-anatomical group characteristics

      b. Growth and developmental patterns

      c. Physiology of skin, hair, and mucus membranes

      d. Diseases more prevalent among group members

      e. Diseases to which the group is relatively resistant

6.   The nurse's assessment, diagnoses, and evaluation of the care outcomes for a minority patient should refelct:

      a. Potential issues involving the interactions between the patient and the elements of the health care system

      b. Problems associated with cultural conflicts between the patient and the health care system

7.   Planning and implementation of care should be adapted as much as possible to the patient's cultural and ethnic background.

Unit 2

SKILLS NECESSARY TO BUILD A FOUNDATION FOR CARE

Basic nursing skills required for establishing a sound foundation for effective patient care are presented in this unit. A foundation composed of a systematic approach to problem solving, the establishment of a functional nurse/patient relationship, the application of principles and techniques of therapeutic communication, and patient advocacy, are essential for planning and implementing effective nursing care. Documentation, recording, and reporting are also critical for maintaining a continuous level of high quality care. Also included in this unit are basic principles of learning and patient teaching. Patient teaching is a significant nursing activity and an integral aspect of patient care. It is a major vehicle for promoting wellness; assisting people to maintain, retain, or restore independence; and for facilitating rehabilitation.

SECTION 1: The Nursing Process

A. Overview of the nursing process

1. The nursing process is a modified scientific approach to problem-solving in the nursing context.

2. The nursing process is a systematic approach to problem-solving used by nurses in all nursing settings with all age groups of patients.

3. The nursing process is a method of organizing, delivering, and evaluating nursing care.

4. The nursing process is a dynamic, open system, continually changing as the patient's problems and nursing care needs change.

5. The nursing process consists of two phases:
    a. Assessment (identifying the problem)
    b. Management (devising a plan of action)

6. The nursing process consists of five steps:
    a. Assessment
    b. Problem identification
    c. Planning
    d. Implementation
    e. Evaluation and modification

7. The strengths of this approach to managing problems encountered in the nursing context are that it involves:
    a. A systematic approach to the problem
    b. Steps in the process which are closely interrelated
    c. A patient-centered approach that allows for active patient participation
    d. Input, throughput, and immediate feedback
    e. An emphasis on the nurse's creativity

8. Limitations to this approach are:
    a. A linear thinking process is implied
    b. An artificial sequence of steps is implied

B. Assessment Phase: Step 1 Assessment

1. Creation of a data base.
    a. Assessment involves the gathering and verification of patient data regarding the patient's level of wellness, risk factors, health practices, health goals, health needs, and patterns of illness.
    b. Nurses gather two types of data:

- Objective data that consist of observations or measurements made by the nurse.
- Subjective data that are patient's perception about their health state and experience.

c. Nurses obtain data from two sources:
  - The primary source of information is the patient.
  - Secondary sources are all other sources of information regarding the patient and their health state, including: family or significant others, neighbors, teachers, health team members, health and personal records, and literature review.

d. Various data gathering methods are used by the nurse during data collection which require the use of cognitive, affective, and/or psychomotor skills.

e. The interview.
  - The interview is the mechanism by which the nurse obtains information regarding the patient's health and physical concerns, observes the patient, and initiates the nurse/patient relationship.
  - There are various interview techniques to use during the interviewing process. These include:
    1. Problem-seeking techinques
    2. Problem-solving techniques
    3. Direct-questioning
    4. Open-ended questioning
  - The basic interview consists of three phases:
    1. The orientation phase
    2. The working phase
    3. The termination phase
  - The interview provides the mechanism for performing the psychosocial examination.

f. The nursing health history.
  - The nursing health history, generally obtained during the initial interview, is the first step in nursing assessment.
  - The health history is data gathered about the patient's level of wellness, changes in life patterns, sociocultural roles, mental and emotional reactions to illness, coping and adaptation skills, and any perceived deviations from normal.
  - Basic components of the nursing health history include:
    1. Biographical information
    2. Reasons for seeking health care
    3. Patient expectations of health care professionals
    4. Past health history

    5. Past history of treatment, hospitalization, outcomes
    6. Family history
    7. Environmental history
    8. Psychosocial history
    9. Present health state and review of symptoms

- The nursing history differs from the medical history in that the *medical* history focuses on the course of the illness/disease process, while the *nursing* history focuses on the degree to which the change in health state has affected the person's ability to meet basic human needs.

g. Physical examination.
- The physical examination uses the skills of measurement, inspection, palpation, percussion, and auscultation to scrutinize all body parts and to verify data gathered during the nursing health history.
- The examination is performed in a systematic manner, usually beginning with data on height, weight, and vital signs, followed by a general survey of the patient's mental status, body development, nutritional status, sex, race, chronological versus apparent age, appearance, and speech, and concludes with a head-to-toe examination of body systems.
- Laboratory and diagnostic tests are used to expand the data base and to verify data gathered through the nursing health history and physical examination. (see Unit 5)

C. Assessment Phase: Step 2 Problem Identification

1. The nursing diagnosis is the end product of the nursing process.

2. A nursing diagnosis is a statement of potential or actual patient problems for which the nurse, by virtue of her/his license and education, is competent to provide intervention.

3. The nursing diagnostic process involves four elements:
    a. Analysis and interpretation of data.
    Interpretation of data requires validation and clustering of salient data. Validation is an ongoing process of determining whether data gathered is complete and accurate.
    b. Clustering of data.
    Clustering of data involves grouping related data, usually signs and symptoms, indicating a general problem.

Data is clustered as it relates to mental or emotional state, individual body systems, risk factors, family data, and/or community factors. As data are clustered, patterns begin to form which help to identify patient's needs, and lead to the formulation of a nursing diagnosis.

c. Identification of patient problems.

An actual health care problem is one that is currently perceived by the patient or assessed by the nurse. A potential health care problem is one for which the patient is at risk. After health care problems are identified, assessment data is refined to support nursing diagnoses.

d. Formulation of nursing diagnosis.
- A nursing diagnosis includes three components.
  1. Statement of the patient's problem.
  2. Statement of causality (etiology).
  3. Signs and symptoms (manifestations), or defining characteristics supporting the nursing diagnosis.
- The problem statement is the current or potential patient problem that can be resolved or mitigated through nursing intervention.
- The statement of causality identifies the focus for the management phase of the nursing care plan.
- The identified signs and symptoms validate the nursing diagnosis.
- Nursing diagnoses are constantly being modified to reflect changing patient needs.

  Example: High risk for infection, (problem identification) related to delayed wound healing (causality) manifested by open gaping wound, and wound healing by secondary intention.

4. Nursing diagnoses are necessary for the formulation of a nursing care plan to help the patient adapt to changes in health state or life-style modifications.

5. Nursing diagnoses help facilitate communication regarding patient care, and can be useful for quality assurance and peer review processes.

6. Errors often identified in formulating nursing diagnoses.

a. Errors of omission involve incomplete assessment, incorrect data clustering, or improper interpretation of data, and result in the failure to accurately identify a problem.

    b. Errors of commission involve the inaccurate data collection and incorrect data clustering, and result in either over-diagnosing or diagnosing nonexistent problems.

    c. Statement errors include:
- The use of inappropriate or imprecise language.
  Example: Fatigue because patient can't rest.
- Stating the nursing diagnosis as a medical diagnosis.
  Example: Diabetes Mellitus
- Using medical terminology to describe the cause of the problem.
  Example: At risk for injury due to Alzheimer's disease.
- Stating the nursing diagnosis as a nursing intervention.
  Example: Nutritional deficit related to need for monitoring dietary intake during meals.
- Stating the diagnosis as a nursing problem.
  Example: At risk for falling related to lack of side rails for the bed.

D. Management Phase: Step 3 Planning

1. Nursing care is individualized care generated and planned around specific nursing diagnoses.

2. A goal is a broad global statement of the desired outcome of nursing interventions.
   Example: The patient will demonstrate knowledge about preventing and detecting infection.

3. Nursing goals include meeting the restorative, rehabilitative, and emergency needs of the patient.

4. Nursing goals are either short-term (achieved quickly), or long-term (achieved sometime in the future).

5. Goals can be prioritized as:
   a. High, reflecting emergency or life-threatening needs
   b. Intermediate, reflecting non-emergency or non-life-threatening needs
   c. Low, reflecting goals not directly related to specific illness or prognosis

6. Objectives are specific directions for how goals can be met. Objectives are stated in measurable terms and contain action verbs. Objectives build in the criteria for evaluating the outcomes of nursing interventions.

> *Example*:   The patient will verbalize the signs and
> symptoms of infection by the second
> hospital day.

7. When prioritizing goals and objectives, the nurse must
consider:
    a. The level of potential patient involvement
    b. Available health care system resources
    c. Limitations imposed by time

8. Nursing interventions, or nursing orders, are planned to reflect
patient care needs, identified goals, and established
objectives. Properly written nursing orders will include:
    a. What is to done
    b. The frequency of the desired actions
    c. The quantity of the desired actions
    d. When the action will be carried out
    e. The method of carrying out the desired actions
    f. Who will carry out the desired actions
        > *Example:*   The nurse will demonstrate the proper
        > technique for effective handwashing
        > before wound care.

9. Improperly written care planning results in incomplete or
inaccurate nursing care, lack of continuity of care, and
the improper use of available resources.

E. Management Phase: Step 4 Implementation

1. Implementation involves taking the nursing actions identified
as necessary to accomplish the designed plan of care.

2. Implementation involves taking actions to:
    a. Assist the patient to accomplish activities of daily living.
    b. Counsel and support the patient and family.
    c. Guide the patient.
    d. Teach the patient, the patient's family, or care giver.
    e. Provide care to achieve the goals of therapy.
    f. Provide an environment conducive to meeting the
    patient's health care needs.

3. Three catagories of nursing interventions have been identified.
    a. Dependent interventions are based upon instructions or
    written directives given by another professional.
        > *Example:*   Administering I.V. antibiotics.
    b. Independent interventions involve aspects of care
    encompassed by licensure and law, requiring no
    directives from others.

> *Example:*   Providing skin care to prevent skin breakdown.
>
> c. Interdependent interventions that nurses carry out in collaboration with another professional.
>
> > *Example:*   Following established protocols for administration of antiarrthythmic drugs in the cardiac care unit.

4. Implementation of the plan of care may require delegation of actions to other personnel whose actions must be evaluated for meeting the standard of care.

5. The care plan is modified as the patient's state of health changes and as needs for care change.

6. The responsibilities of the nurse in implementing the patient's plan of care include:
   a. Reviewing planned interventions
   b. Scheduling patient activities
   c. Collaborating with members of the health care team
   d. Providing direct care
   e. Supervising direct care actions delegated to others
   f. Counseling patients and staff
   g. Teaching patient, family, or substitute care giver
   h. Making appropriate referrals
   i. Documenting and maintaining patient records

F. Management Phase: Step 5 Evaluation and Modification

1. Documentation and reporting the evaluation of the care plan is an obligation of professional accountability.

2. Evaluation is conducted to determine the degree to which goals and objectives have been achieved and to judge the effectiveness of the nursing care plan.

3. The evaluation process involves five steps:
   a. Establishing individualized evaluation criteria based upon projected outcomes
   b. Comparing the patient's responses to the established criteria
   c. Analyzing variables affecting intervention outcomes
   d. Identifying reasons for failure to achieve desired outcomes
   e. Taking corrective actions to modify the nursing care plan

4. Evaluation is a continuous process that determines the quality of care.

5. Factors that can influence the outcomes of care include:

     a. Current, accurate, and complete assessment of data

     b. Correct analysis of health care needs

     c. Correctly identifying problem and causality

     d. Realistic short and long term goals and objectives

     e. Effectiveness and efficiency of nursing actions

     f. Available resources and personnel

6. Modification of the plan of care plan is based upon the conclusions developed during evaluation of the projected outcomes.

7. Modification of the care plan, to reflect current patient needs and determine the degree of problem resolution, is the most often overlooked and neglected aspect of the nursing process.

8. Modification of the plan of care may involve reassessment and/or replanning.

9. The nurse must implement the modified plan of care and re-evaluate the patient's response to that plan.

10. Health care agencies often use the evaluation process to establish their own systems for identifying, examining, or verifying nursing care (nursing audit).

11. Evaluation of the care plan and outcomes of nursing interventions may be used for:

     a. Malpractice suits

     b. Staff evaluations, reviews, or promotions

     c. Nursing research

     d. Quality improvement

G. Quality improvement

1. Quality improvement focuses on the evaluation and improvement of the delivery of care.

2. Terms currently used to refer to quality improvement include:

     a. (Total quality management (T.Q.M.)

     b. Continuous quality improvement (C.Q.I.).

3. Quality improvement is based on the assumption that processes can always be improved, and involves:

     a. A systematic approach to balancing an increasing effectiveness of organization against cost reduction methods

     b. A continuous evaluation of the needs and expectations of those who consume services and how to meet those needs more efficiently (patient satisfaction)

     c. A long-term commitment to the organization's philosophy

SECTION 2: Communication Skills

A. Communication skills in nursing

1.   Individuals have a need to relate their ideas, thoughts, and emotions to others in a meaningful way.

2.   The ability to communicate effectively is an essential component of nursing practice and the delivery of total health care.

3.   Communication is a complex process requiring the application of principles that involve the transmission of mutually negotiated meanings and symbols between and among individuals.

4.   Communication in nursing provides the foundation for the establishment of the nurse/patient relationship and a means to effect change.

B. Factors influencing communication

1.   To be effective the receiver must perceive the sender's message accurately.

2.   Intrapersonal variables that can influence the accuracy of communication messages are:
   a.   Perceptions, or personal view and interpretation, of events occurring around the individual.
   b.   Values, personal beliefs, and convictions regarding certain ideas and behaviors.
   c.   Emotions or subjective feelings about the events occurring around the individual.
   d.   Sociocultural background, or cultural frame of reference, that forms the individual's generalizations and preconceptions about the world.
   e.   Knowledge and developmental level that influences vocabulary use and words chosen to express ideas.
   f.   Roles and relationships perceived to exist among individuals in dialogue.
   g.   Environmental setting in which the communication occurs.

3.   Effective messages are clear, concise, organized, and expressed in a manner familiar to the individual receiving the message.

C. Levels of communication

1. Communication are interpersonal and intrapersonal interactions that occur on a social level for the purpose of sharing information.
2. Communication can occur on three levels.
   a. Intrapersonal communication occurring within an individual.
   b. Interpersonal communication occurring between two people or in small groups.
   c. Public communication involving interaction in large groups of people.
3. Individuals may or may not be aware of the elements of communication.

D. The communication process

1. The nurse needs to develop an awareness of the elements of communication, and must know how to analyze each element of the communication process. This is essential in order to control interactions effectively.
2. Elements of the communication process include:
   a. The referent (factor that motivates a person to communicate)
   b. The sender (one who initiates the communication)
   c. The message (information sent or expressed by the sender)
   d. The channels (means of conveying messages)
   e. The receiver (person to whom the information is sent)
   f. Feedback (information that serves to reveal whether the meaning of the sender's message was received)
3. Information and meaning can be lost or gained if any element of the process is altered.

E. Types of communication

1. Communication can be natural, uninhibited, or consciously manipulated.
2. Verbal communication
   a. Verbal communication involves the written or spoken word.
   b. Words can be of two types of meaning:
      • Denotative meanings are those shared by individuals who use a common language.
      • Connotative meanings are those apart from what is explicitly described as a word's meaning.

      c. Communication is more successful when a verbal message is appropriately paced.

      d. The speaker's tone can convey the meaning and mood of a verbal message.

      e. Clarity and brevity can enhance communication and decrease distortion of verbal messages.

      f. Timing and relevance are elements influencing the reception of verbal messages.

3. Nonverbal communication is the transmission of messages without the use of words.

      a. We communicate non-verbally in every face-to-face encounter.

      b. Nonverbal cues add meaning to what is communicated verbally.

      c. Nonverbal cues can repeat what is being said verbally.

      d. Nonverbal cues can emphasize the spoken word.

      e. Nonverbal cues can substitute for words.

      f. Verbal and nonverbal messages can contradict each other.

      g. There are various channels for communicating nonverbally:
- Appearance
- Facial expression
- Posture and gait
- Hand gestures
- Touch
- Space and territoriality

F. Therapeutic communication

1. Social interactions, unlike therapeutic interactions, are superficial in nature. In the nursing context, they constitute early attempts to communicate with a patient.

2. Several relationship types comprise the nurse/patient relationship.

      a. The goal of the nurse is to help the patient develop a sense of trust in the relationship so that the patient will feel comfortable discussing attitudes, feelings, and concerns.

      b. The therapeutic nurse/patient relationship is a "time limited" relationship; there is a specific beginning and end to the relationship.

      c. Therapeutic relationships are formed for a specific purpose.

    d. Therapeutic relationships facilitate physical and psychological support, growth, and change in the patient.

3. Three growth facilitating conditions essential to the development and maintenance of a therapeutic relationship are:
    a. Genuineness (being real)
    b. Empathy ("feeling with" versus "feeling for")
    c. Unconditional positive regard (acceptance)

4. Characteristics of a helping relationship include:
    a. Trust
    b. Empathy
    c. Sympathy
    d. Caring
    e. Autonomy
    f. Mutuality

5. Phases of the therapeutic nurse/patient relationship are:
    a. Pre-encounter
      • Period to review patient information prior to meeting with the patient and to plan for the interview

    b. Orientation phase
      • The primary objective of this phase is building trust.
      • Problems and goals are identified.
      • Roles and expectations are clarified.
      • Contracts are formed.

    c. Working phase
      • The primary objective of this phase is problem mitigation, or resolution, and effecting change.
      • Valuable action-oriented communication strategies used during this phase include:
        1. Immediacy in communication
        2. Sensitive confrontation
        3. Concreteness in communication

    d. Termination phase
      • Because the nurse patient relationship is a time limited relationship, the termination phase ideally begins during the orientation phase.
      • The primary objective of this phase is separation from the relationship in a mutually planned and satisfying manner.
      • The patient and nurse evaluate the degree to which the goals of the relationship have been achieved.

- Termination can be stressful and painful for the patient and for the nurse.

G. Effective communication techniques

1. Maintain silence to facilitate the organization of thoughts, the processing of information, and intrapersonal communication.

2. Listen attentively to perceive the complete meaning of the communication and analyze the message.
   a. Face the speaker.
   b. Maintain eye contact.
   c. Assume a relaxed, open posture.
   d. Lean toward the speaker.
   e. Nod appropriately.
   f. Avoid distracting movements.

3. Convey acceptance by:
   a. Listening without interruption
   b. Providing verbal feedback
   c. Matching verbal and nonverbal cues
   d. Avoiding argument, expressing doubt, or attempting to change the patient's mind

4. Ask questions to elicit specific information, selecting logical questions based on the patient's previous response.
   a. Open-ended questions elicit bredth of information.
      Example: Tell me more about your daughter.
   b. Closed-ended questions elicit a narrow, specific response.
      Example: How old is your daughter?

5. Paraphrase the patient's message.

6. Clarify messages to verify meaning, increase understanding, and reduce misunderstandings.

7. Keep the interaction focused to limit the areas of discussion, reduce vagueness, and deepen the level of communication.

8. One way to provide feedback to the patient regarding messages is to comment on the patient's behavior.

9. Offering information encourages the patient to respond further, based on the nurse's input, and can help with the decision-making process.

10. Summarizing is a concise way to review of the key ideas that have been discussed. It helps to convey meaning and understanding of messages and sets the tone for further communication.

11. Be willing to engage in selective self-disclosure when appropriate.

H. **Barriers to effective communication**

1. Avoid giving opinions that transfer decision-making to the nurse and prevent the patient from solving his or her problems.

2. Avoid giving false reassurance as an attempt to reduce patient fear and anxiety.

3. Avoid being defensive or conveying the impression that the patient is not free to express an opinion.

4. Avoid communicating signs of approval and/or disapproval.

5. Avoid asking "Why" since it causes feelings of resentment, insecurity, and mistrust in the patient.

6. Avoid inappropriate shifts in topic since they retard the progress of therapeutic communication. This may also imply disinterest or convey a lack of attention on the part of the nurse.

I. **Communicating with children**

1. Communication with infants occurs primarily on a nonverbal level.

2. When communicating with infants, avoid loud hard sounds, use close physical contact, and keep the mother, or care giver, in the infant's line of view when interacting with the child.

3. Toddlers and preschoolers communicate verbally and nonverbally, and their speech is concrete.

4. When communicating with toddler and preschoolers, focus on their personal needs and concerns using simple, short sentences, familiar words, and concrete explanations.

5. School-age children's communication is primarily verbal.

6. When communicating with school-age children, give simple explanations and encourage expressions of feelings and concerns.

7. Adolescents think on a more abstract level.

8. When communicating with adolescents, avoid imposing values or judgments that show disapproval, and avoid interrupting.

9. Use attentive listening skills and constantly clarify terms.

SECTION 3: Basics Of Recording And Reporting

A. Recording and Reporting

1. Reports and records provide a mechanism for communicating specific information regarding a patient's overall condition and response to medical therapy and nursing care interventions.

2. The patient's record is a permanent document important to health care management.

3. The patient's chart is a legal document and should contain only factual, patient information.

4. Legal guidelines for charting deal with *how* to document rather than *what* to document.

5. The chart belongs to the health care agency but the information within the chart belongs to the patient.

B. Purposes of record keeping in health care

1. Each facility uses its own recording format but all charts contain basic information.
   a. Demographic data
   b. Consent forms
   c. Admission histories: nursing and medical
   d. Reports of physical and diagnostic examinations
   e. Patient's nursing and medical diagnoses
   f. Therapeutic orders
   g. Progress notes
   h. Nursing care plans
   i. Record of care, treatments and patient teaching
   j. Discharge summary and plan

2. Purposes of maintaining patient records.
   a. Facilitating communication among health care providers
   b. Facilitating care planning
   c. Organizing patient educational needs
   d. Generating a data base and facilitating evaluation of the patient's progress
   e. Auditing and monitoring care
   f. Providing research data
   g. Providing legal documentation of the patient's course of treatment and care

3. Types of records.

  a. Source-oriented records filed according to type of care giver
  b. Problem-oriented medical records (POMR) filed according to problems identified.
  c. Computer generated documentation
  d. Flow sheets that make recording quicker, less redundant, and are used to visually display patient data over time

C. Characteristics of professional recording and reporting

  1. Information must represent a correct, objective interpretation of patient data with precise measurements, correct spellings, and proper use of terminology and abbreviations.

  2. Nurses report and record their own observations or measurements, not what they think might have happened or information given to them by other nurses.

  3. Nonessential information, that which can be misleading or confusing, should be omitted from reports and recordings.

  4. Proper reporting is concise, thorough, and incorporates all relevant patient information.

  5. Reported information is organized logically in the order of occurrence and documented in a timely manner. Changes in a patient's condition are reported and recorded immediately.

  6. There are laws protecting information gathered about patients and their course of care. Nurses are responsible for keeping patient information confidential.

  7. The chart should accompany the patient in the hospital or clinic at all times and the staff should be aware of the whereabouts of the patient's record at all times.

  8. Legibility is essential, especially when recording numbers and medical terminology.

  9. Nurses must be familiar with, and correctly use:
  a. Commonly used descriptive charting terms
  b. Commonly used approved abbreviations
  c. Commonly used combining forms (prefixes and suffixes)

D. Reporting

  1. Change-of shift reporting.
  a. Continuity of patient care between nurses is maintained by the change-of-shift report.

  b. Change-of-shift reports are given verbally, in person, or on audio tape.

  c. An organized presentation saves time, is efficient, and reduces the omission of relevant patient information.

  d. Below is a suggested organization for change-of-shift report.
- Patient name, age, sex
- Diagnoses; nursing and medical
- Description of physiological and psychological conditions
- Scheduled tests, procedures or surgeries, and the patient's psychological responses or concerns regarding tests, procedures, or surgeries
- Modification in therapy
- Modification in diet or fluid restriction
- Significant medications and the effects of those medications on the patient
- Responses of the patient to nursing care interventions and patient progress toward established long- and short-term goals
- Patient teaching; planned projects and completed projects
- Significant information regarding the family or social network
- Significant changes in the patient's condition and priority situations for the oncoming nursing team

2. Nursing rounds.

  a. Nursing rounds are used for change-of-shift report, care planning, and education.

  b. The nurse assigned to the patient summarizes the patient's current status and care plan.

  c. Nursing rounds facilitate optimal nurse communication and direct patient observation.

  d. Nursing rounds encourage collaborative efforts for patient care and problem solving, and facilitates the immediate discussion of nursing and patient issues.

3. Telephone reporting.

  a. Information regarding the patient is often communicated by telephone.

  b. Telephone communications regarding the patient's condition or other relevant patient information must always be recorded in the patient's chart.

  c. Telephone reports must always be verified. This can be accomplished by having the receiver repeat messages clearly and precisely back to the sender.

E. Computerization of health care records

1. Computers are now commonplace in health care settings.

2. Bedside computers offer a number of advantages to the nursing team for recording and communicating patient information.

3. Computerized decision-making support systems may become available to assist nurses in professional decision-making and care planning.

4. Computerized record systems have the advantage of being more organized, legible, accessible, and comprehensive.

5. Computerized systems may be helpful for improving clinical decisions and judgments in novice and beginning level nurses.

F. Reporting and recording in the home health setting

1. Comprehensively and objectively document the specific reasons the client is homebound.

2. Document complications related to the client's diagnoses.

3. Describe skilled nursing care received including observation, assessment, teaching, and case management issues.

4. Document the continuing need for skilled nursing care.

5. When recording self-care skills taught to clients, explain the degree of assistance necessary to perform skill correctly.

6. Document all identified learning needs, knowledge deficits, and continuing need for patient teaching.

G. Incident reports

1. Incident reports are filed when something occurs that could, or actually did, cause injury or that was not good care.

2. Incident reports are used by agency administration for purposes of quality assurance and risk management.

3. Typical unusual occurrences requiring an incident report include:
   a. Medication errors
   b. Patient falls
   c. Patient injuries
   d. Staff injuries

4. Incident reports can be used to:
   a. Identify areas of client risk
   b. Assess potential liability and future insurance claims

    c. Suggest areas for staff education and development

5. Incident reports are the property of the hospital and are considered privileged information between the agency and, in most states, its legal representative.

SECTION 4: Basic Principles of the Teaching-Learning Process

A. The purpose of patient teaching

1. Teaching is a deliberate and conscious process that promotes learning.

2. Teaching prepares people to perform new functions and solve problems.

3. Teaching is most effective when it meets the learner's need and desire for information and knowledge.

4. Learning is a process of acquiring new knowledge or skills through practice and reinforcement.

5. Teaching is a form of communication, and the steps of the teaching process are similar to the nursing process.
   a. Assess the patient's learning needs.
   b. Identify knowledge deficits.
   c. Establish a teaching plan.
      • Establish a goal for the teaching plan.
      • Establish learning objectives for accomplishing the goal.
   d. Implement the teaching plan.
   e. Evaluate the effectiveness of the teaching plan.

6. Nurses are responsible for assessing a patient's learning needs, providing information, and thereby helping patients to increase their ability to function and maintain independence.

7. Patient teaching facilitates several important patient goals.
   a. To maintain good health and health habits
   b. To prevent illness, disease, and injury
   c. To restore and regain health or impaired functioning
   d. To develop coping strategies to deal with impaired functioning or permanent disability
   e. To prevent patient complications
   f. To increase adherence to treatment regimes

8. Every encounter between the nurse and the patient provides an opportunity for health teaching.

B. Domains of learning

1. There are three principle domains of learning behavior.
   a. Cognitive behaviors that include intellectual activities such as comprehension, application, analysis, synthesis, and evaluation.
   Example: The patient will explain the relationship between exercise and dietary intake.
   b. Affective behaviors that include dealing with feelings related to attitudes, opinions, or values.
   Example: The patient will explore the possible source of her anxiety.
   c. Psychomotor behaviors that include the acquisition of skills requiring integration of mental and muscular activities
   Example: The patient will demonstrate the ability to self-inject Insulin.
2. Teaching specific behaviors will often involve incorporating behaviors from all three domains.
3. An effective and comprehensive teaching plan will include behaviors from all of the identified domains.

C. Basic learning principles

1. Effective teaching requires the use of strategies by which a patient learns best.
2. The patient's ability to learn will depend on three conditions.
   a. The patient's readiness to learn, which depends on:
      - Attention set
      - Level of motivation
      - Health beliefs
      - Desire to learn

   b. The patient's ability to learn, which depends on:
      - Physical and cognitive capabilities
      - Developmental level
      - Physical wellness.
      - Cognitive functioning and degree of organization

   c. The learning environment, which includes:
      - The number of persons being taught at one time
      - Privacy
      - Room temperature and ventilation
      - Lighting

- Noise level
- Internal and external distractions
- Room furnishings
- Educational materials available in the language read by the patient and/or care givers.

D. Basic teaching principles

1. An effective teacher schedules the teaching activities at times when the patient is most receptive and alert.

2. The organization of the content in a presentation should progress from simple, concrete ideas to more complex, or abstract, ideas.

3. Teaching strategies should encourage and maximize active learner participation.

4. Teaching is most effective when it builds upon the learner's existing knowledge base.

5. Teaching strategies should match the learner's type of learning need.

6. Learning objectives are written in behavioral terms that anticipate what the patient will learn.

7. An effective teaching plan is mutually established by the nurse, patient, and care givers to define the information and skills necessary to increase independence.

8. An effective teaching plan takes into consideration the patient's cognitive abilities and limitations.

SECTION 5: Ethics In Nursing

A. Definition of ethics

1. Ethics are principles or standards that dictate conduct.

2. Moral beliefs are convictions regarding absolute right and wrong.

3. Ethical rights indicate how people "ought" to act but involve no legal guarantee.

4. Ethical, moral, and legal issues are frequently confused; however, they are not necessarily the same things.

5. The complex and highly technical nature of the current health care system has meant increasing exposure of nurses to ethical dilemmas.

B. Professional ethics

1. The American Nurses' Association developed a Code of Ethics in 1976.

2. Each nurse is responsible for the scope of functions and duties associated with the nurse's role in providing patient care.

3. Accountability is being answerable for one's actions.

4. Accountability applies to the entire scope of functions and duties nurses are required to perform.

5. The nurse is accountable to his or her self, to the patient, to the employing institution, and to society for the effectiveness of care provided.

6. Accountability serves four basic purposes:
   a. Evaluation and reassessment of professional practices
   b. Maintaining standards of care
   c. Facilitating personal reflection and growth
   d. Providing a basis for ethical decision making

7. Nurses must be actively involved in ethical decision-making.

C. Nursing advocacy

1. Advocacy in nursing is a complex process of providing patients with accurate information, protecting patients' rights, and supporting patients' decisions.

2. The process of advocacy requires that the nurse understand his or her own attitudes, values, and beliefs.

3. Having knowledge of themselves, nurses can better recognize and accept the idea that a patient's values, beliefs, and attitudes may be different.

4. The nurse advocate may have to consider the patient's desire for information while being careful not to interfere with the patient's relationships with other professionals and family members.

5. Decision-making is the responsibility of the patient. The nurse advocate must support the patient in decision-making without becoming defensive or placing his or her self in the rescuing position.

6. The nurse advocate refrains from giving advice, offering opinions, being judgmental, or offering approval or disapproval.

7. The only time patients should be omitted from decision-making is when they are in a state of total dependency.

D. Ethical dilemmas

1. Ethical issues can arise from five entities of nursing accountability:
   a. The self
   b. The client
   c. The profession
   d. The Institution
   e. Society

2. Ethical dilemmas encountered in nursing practice often involve principles of truth telling, loyalty, felicity towards others, and self-determination.

3. Patient-centered dilemmas often involve issues of:
   a. Abortion
   b. Behavioral control
   c. Rights to health care
   d. Definitions of death.

4. Nurse-physician-patient dilemmas often involve issues related to:
   a. Confidentiality
   b. Informed consent
   c. Role conflict.

5. Nurse-co-worker dilemmas often involve issues related to:
   a. Interdependent relationships
   b. Maintaining ethical standards
   c. Common licensure

E. Ethical dilemma resolution process

1. No ethical dilemma will be resolved easily, nor will two ethical dilemmas ever be exactly the same.

2. Sound, ethical decisions are made using careful judgment and a methodological decision-making approach.

3. A proposed method for approaching ethical dilemmas involve specific deliberate actions.
   a. An initial recognition occurs that a dilemma exists ("I ought to").
   b. Relevant information related to the issue is collected

   c. Emotions, attitudes, or values influencing perceptions of the dilemma are identified
   d. Ethical principles related to the dilemma (i.e. truth telling) are identified
   e. Analysis of the dilemma includes idientification of:
- Who is involved in the dilemma?
- What are the implications of the dilemma?
- What are the consequences of all alternatives, choices, or solutions that could be taken?
- Outcomes of action or choices are evaluated

   f. The action/solution is acted upon.

Unit 3

BASIC HUMAN NEEDS

uman beings are individuals with biological and psychological needs for maintaining life and well-being. Nursing is the art and science of helping persons to meet those essential requirements, preventing the development of unmet needs and problems, and maintaining an optimal level of independence. This chapter discusses the use of a human needs approach in the organization of patient care. Maslow's five categories of human needs are presented. Various obstacles that can interfere in the satisfaction of needs are identified. Characteristic indicators of unmet needs, and the suggested basic nursing measures to assist the patient in meeting needs are given. Although the discussion of various needs suggests that they are unrelated, in practice they are highly related.

SECTION 1: A Basic Human Needs Approach to Patient Care

A. Basic human needs

1. Basic human needs include the necessities of survival and health.
2. Basic needs can be prioritized along levels of need.
3. Developmental stage and state of health influence the individual's ability to meet needs without assistance.
4. One way to represent, evaluate, and understand basic needs is given by Maslow's hierarchy of needs.
5. Individual needs may be totally met, partially met, or unmet.
6. A person's state of health and wellness is significantly influenced by his or her ability to meet basic needs.
7. Patients entering the health care setting who require nursing care usually have unmet needs or are no longer able to meet their needs independently.
8. Human needs theory can:
   a. Provide a foundation for nursing care
   b. Apply to persons in all developmental stages
   c. Provide concepts important for understanding health and illness
   d. Provide a scheme for prioritizing patient problems and nursing care issues

B. Basic human needs

1. Physiological needs
2. Safety needs
3. Love and affection needs
4. Esteem needs
5. Self-actualization needs

C. Barriers to meeting human needs

1. Various factors encountered in everyday living can act as barriers to meeting needs.
2. Physiological barriers:
   a. Illness
   b. Fatigue
   c. Pain

    d. Immobility

    e. Physical limitation

3. Emotional barriers:
   a. Anxiety
   b. Excitement
   c. Fear
   d. Frustration

4. Social barriers:
   a. Strained personal relationships
   b. Feelings of insecurity
   c. Feelings of inadequacy
   d. Feelings of intimidation
   e. Inadequate social network
   f. Sense of isolation

5. Intellectual barriers:
   a. Lack of information
   b. Lack of knowledge
   c. Lack of understanding
   d. Cognitive dysfunction or disorganization

6. Environmental barriers:
   a. Extremes in environmental conditions
   b. Unfamiliar surroundings
   c. Unsafe living conditions
   d. Pollution

7. Cultural barriers:
   a. Values
   b. Beliefs
   c. Practices
   d. Habits
   e. Life-style choices

8. Situations resulting in unmet needs or partially met needs can create a state of dis-ease or disequalibrium within the person.

D. Application of needs theory

1. To be most effective in planning care for patients, the nurse must understand the interrelatedness of basic human needs.

2. It is also important to understand the underlying factors that determine the priority needs for each person.

3. Nursing care involves taking a holistic view of the person and this often involves meeting many human needs simultaneously.

4. It is often necessary for nursing to prioritize patient needs so that care can be focused and effective.
   a. Life threatening situations always take priority.
      Example: Meeting oxygen needs for a child with an airway obstruction.
   b. Unmet physiological needs posing a threat to life have high priority.
      Example: Meeting nutritional needs for a cancer patient receiving chemotherapy.
   c. Some needs must be deferred until the patient's health state stabilizes or improves.
      Example: Meeting belonging needs for a patient being stabilized following head trauma.
   d. Family patterns and habits should be considered when prioritizing care aimed at assisting patients in meeting needs.
   e. A patient's perception of need varies and this should be considered when prioritizing a plan to assist in meeting needs.
   f. In some situations the care can be adjusted to correspond to the patient's personality and mood.

SECTION 2: Physiological Needs

A. Physiological needs

1. Meeting physiological needs is a fundamental human drive and of the five basic needs, it is given highest priority.

2. Oxygen.
   a. The body depends on oxygen for existence and metabolic processes.
   b. Oxygen must be supplied from the environment to the lung, the blood stream, and the tissues.
   c. The body does not maintain an oxygen reserve and so requires a constant supply.
   d. The functions of the respiratory system are oxygen intake, gas exchange, and carbon dioxide elimination.
   e. Indicators of inadequate oxygenation include:
      • Confusion
      • Lethargy

- Air hunger
- Restlessness
- Nasal flaring
- Sternal, substernal and suprasternal flaring
- Rapid, shallow respiration
- Cyanosis of the skin and mucous membranes
- Alterations in blood gases

   f. Nursing measures to assist in the meeting of oxygen needs include:
- Cardiopulmonary resuscitation
- Maintaining an open airway
- Suctioning to remove obstructive secretions
- Maintaining adequate hydration
- Mobilizing secretions
- Positive-pressure breathing (IPPB)
- Positioning to facilitate lung expansion
- Administering oxygen therapy
- Reducing anxiety
- Chest physiotherapy
  1. Postural drainage
  2. Percussion
  3. Vibration
- Nebulization
- Administering medications
- Mechanical ventilation

3. Fluids.
   a. The body must maintain a balance between fluids taken in and those excreted.
   b. Fluids may be taken into the body by oral or parenteral routes and are removed from the body through the lungs, intestines, skin, and kidneys.
   c. Patients who are very young, very elderly, severely ill, or acutely traumatized are at highest risk in adequate fluid balance.
   d. Water is the main constituent of body fluid. Water and electrolytes are distributed between the intracellular and extracellular fluid.
   e. Conditions resulting from inadequate fluid maintenance are:
- Dehydration, the excessive loss of water from body tissues
- Edema, the abnormal accumulation of fluids in interstitial spaces, the peritoneal cavity, or joint capsules.
   f. Dehydration may result from:
- Vomiting

- Diarrhea
- Rapid fluid loss (i.e. burns)
- Altered level of consciousness
- Inability to take fluids orally
- Prolonged fever

g. Indicators of dehydration include:
- Electrolyte imbalance
- Poor skin turgor
- Flushed, dry skin
- Decreased tearing, salivating, or sweating
- Coated tongue
- Oliguria
- Urinary tract irritability, incontinence, or infection
- Irritability
- Confusion
- Severe dehydration coma

h. Edema may result from:
- Nutritional disorders
- Cardiovascular disorders
- Renal disorders
- Hepatic disease
- Trauma
- Water intoxication
- Drug administration

i. Indicators of edema include:
- Presence of fluid in the tissues of the extremities, periorbital areas, sacral area assessed by light palpation and graded 1+ to 4+ severity
- Smooth, shiny skin susceptible to breakdown
- Presence of ascites
- Daily weight gain
- Shortness of breath
- Increased heart rate
- Complaints of tight shoes or rings
- Altered level of consciousness

j. Nursing measures to assist in the meeting of fluid needs include:
- Maintaining adequate fluid intake, normally 2600 ml per day.
- Restoring fluid balance
- Restoring electrolyte balance
- Restoring acid-base balance
- Treating underlying conditions creating the imbalance
- Taking measures to protect the skin and underlying tissues

- Providing a safe environment for the patient with altered level of consciousness of confusion
- Monitoring intake and output

4. Nutrition.
   a. The body requires nutrients, minerals, and vitamins to maintain its demands for energy.
   b. The body's metabolic processes control digestion, storage, and elimination of digestive waste products from the body.
   c. Digestive processes break down nutrients into usable compounds:
      - Those meeting immediate energy needs, glucose, and amino acids
      - Those stored for later use as glycogen, protein, fat
   d. Each individual has a therapeutic calorie demand to meet his or her energy needs. Caloric intake greater than bodily need results in being overweight, and a caloric intake less than bodily needs results in being underweight.
   e. A variety of biological, psychological, social, and cultural factors influence dietary pattern and status.
   f. Indicators of inadequate nutrition can include:
      - Failure to maintain ideal body weight
      - Failure to grow
      - Unplanned weight loss
      - Fatigue
      - Pallor
      - Recurring sores in the mouth and on the gums
      - Brittle hair and nails
   g. Nursing measures to assist in the meeting of nutrition needs include:
      - Monitoring food intake pattern
      - Monitoring weight
      - Teaching nutrition
      - Providing supplements
      - Providing an appetizing dining environment
      - Maintaining nutrition when gastrointestinal function is impaired

5. Temperature.
   a. The body can function normally between a narrow temperature range, but temporarily can regulate temperature outside that range.
   b. Patients can experience conditions related to both heat and cold. A rapid change in temperature, exposure to

extreme temperatures, or inability to regulate temperature can result in severe illness or death.
  c. Body temperature is a frequently used indicator of health and illness.
  d. Indicators of prolonged exposure to cold can include:
    • Decreased rate of metabolism
    • Decrease oxygen consumption
    • Decrease in vital signs
    • Alteration in level of consciousness
    • Pale and cold skin
    • Decreased urinary output
    • Frostbite of exposed areas

  e. Indicators of prolonged exposure to heat can include:
    • Increased metabolic rate
    • Increased oxygen demand and consumption
    • Local exposure to heat resulting in first, second, and third degree burns
    • Over exposure to the sun causing sun stroke involving high fever, seizures, and coma
    • Over exposure to hot weather resulting in heatstroke involving fever, dehydration, fluid and electrolyte imbalance, confusion, and coma

  f. Nursing measures to assist in the meeting of temperature needs include:
    • Restoring normal body temperature
      1. Administering antipyretic drugs
      2. Tepid water baths
      3. Maintaining adequate nutrition
      4. Maintaining adequate hydration
      5. Promoting rest and sleep
    • Restoring body temperature regulation
    • Identifying risk factors for extreme temperature exposure
    • Treating frostbite
    • Emergency treatment for sun stroke
    • Treating heat stroke
    • Treating burns
    • Monitoring body temperature
    • Providing shelter from the elements

6. Elimination.
  a. Waste materials from ingested food are eliminated by the lungs, skin, kidneys, and the intestines.
  b. The lungs primarily eliminate CO_2 and water (200 ml/day) on expiration.

    c. The skin eliminates water (200 ml/day) and sodium in the form of sweat.

    d. The kidneys depend on fluid intake and circulatory blood volume to eliminate excess body fluid, electrolytes, hydrogen ions and acids in the urine.

    e. The intestines eliminate solid waste products and some fluid from the body.

    f. Indicators of inadequate elimination can include:
- Urinary incontinence
- Fluid and electrolyte imbalances
- Dehydration
- Edema
- Changes in elimination pattern
- Constipation
- Diarrhea

    g. Nursing measures to assist in the meeting of elimination needs include:
- Providing assistance in meeting elimination needs
  1. Stimulating bowel elimination
  2. Preventing and managing constipation
  3. Reducing flatulence
- Monitoring diet and fluid intake
- Bowel and bladder training
- Ostomy care
- Urinary catheterization
- Bladder irrigation

7. Shelter.

    a. The body requires shelter from the environmental elements.

    b. Indicators of inadequate shelter can include:
- Exposure to temperature extremes
- Residence in unsafe housing and neighborhoods
- Limited financial, social, and family resources
- Living in environments subject to exposure to dirt, vermin, or insects
- Poorly lighted or cluttered environments.

    c. Nursing measures to assist in the meeting of shelter needs include:
- Referral to community agencies
- Modifying the home environment to reduce risk factors
- Patient teaching regarding the home and work environment, and health promotion

8. Rest.

    a. Every individual has a physiological need for rest and sleep which varies, depending on:

- Age
- Activity pattern
- Health status
- Life-style
- Quality of rest and sleep
- Physical and emotional stress levels

b. Sleep is a cyclic phenomenon composed of two distinct types of activity:
  - Rapid eye movement, about 25 per cent of nightly sleep
  - Non-rapid eye movement, about 75 per cent of nightly sleep

c. Alterations in sleep pattern include:
  - Excessive somnolence
  - Narcolepsy
  - Sleep apnea
  - Insomnia
  - Restless leg syndrome

d. Common barriers to meeting rest needs include:
  - Life-style
  - Work schedule
  - Temporary activities
  - Disturbance in normal sleep pattern
  - Disruption to bed time routine
  - Pain
  - Sensory deprivation and sensory overload
  - Stress

e. Indicators of inadequate rest can include:
  - Decreased energy
  - Disheveled appearance
  - Circles under the eyes
  - Decreased motivation
  - Decreased concentration and attention span
  - Irritability
  - Restlessness
  - Withdrawal behaviors
  - Falling asleep during the day
  - Hallucinations (in severe cases)

f. Nursing measures to assist in the meeting of rest needs include:
  - Attempts to maintain normal sleep-wake cycle
  - Attempts to maintain bedtime routine
  - Scheduling rest periods
  - Providing appropriate level of activity and diversion

- Providing adequate pain control and management
- Identifying and attempting to resolve underlying cause of sleep disturbance such as life style issues or chronic stress

9. Sex.
   a. Sex is a basic physiological need influenced by age, sociocultural background, ethics, values, self-esteem, and health status.
   b. Sexuality is more than physical sexual activity, it involves emotional, social and spiritual needs.
   c. The meeting of sexual needs can be influenced by illness, chronic condition, and hospitalization.
   d. Indicators that patients are having difficulty meeting sexual needs include:
      - Excessive sexual or suggestive language
      - Excessive masturbation
      - Exposing external sexual organs
      - Flirting
      - Sublimation through excessive physical exercise, overwork, or overeating
      - Showing signs of stress and frustration
   e. Common barriers to meeting sexual needs include:
      - Lack of privacy
      - Chronic debilitating illness or conditions
      - Alteration in body image and reduced sense of confidence as a sexual being
      - Depression
      - Grieving
      - Life-style changes
      - Puberty
      - Pregnancy
      - Menopause
   f. Nursing measures to assist the patient in meeting sexual needs must be individualized based upon the patient's age, maturity, sexual partner, sexual practices, and degree of comfort in discussing sexuality.
   g. The PLISSIT model of progressive intervention is the accepted model for intervening in altered sexuality.

Stage 1 P -	permission given to talk about sexual concerns
Stage 2 LI -	sharing factual knowledge about sexuality
Stage 3 SS -	providing specific information to prevent or alleviate specific sexual problems
Stage 4 IT -	intensive therapy with a qualified therapist

SECTION 3: Safety and Security Needs

A. Safety and security needs

1. Second-level needs involve those of physical and psychological safety and security.

2. As individuals grow and develop, their dependence for meeting basic human needs gradually decreases until they can generally function independently.

3. Illness, physical and mental challenges, and hospitalization can restrict a person's ability to meet his or her needs for physical safety without assistance.
   a. Meeting physical safety needs involves reducing or eliminating threats to life and well-being.
   b. When assessing the patient's total environment for physical safety threats, actual and potential hazards must be considered.
   c. Threats to physical safety include:
      - Immobility
      - Medication therapy
      - Altered states of consciousness
      - Decreased sensory modality acuity
      - Problems with balance and stability
      - Invasive therapeutic procedures
      - Risk-taking behavior
      - Occupational hazards
      - Unsound health practices
      - Unsafe life choices
      - Isolated lifestyle
      - Emotional stress

   d. Nursing measures to assist patients in meeting physical safety needs include:
      - Identifying actual dangers
      - Identifying potential risk factors
      - Teaching patient regarding safety issues of childhood
      - Teaching patient regarding identified hazards
      - Teaching patient regarding medication therapy

4. Psychological safety and security comes from one's ability to:
   a. Predict other people's behaviors
   b. Understanding the expectations of others
   c. Predicting conditions in the environment

5. Everyone feels threatened when exposed to new, unexpected, or unfamiliar surroundings or events.

6. Indicators that a patient may be experiencing a threat are usually demonstrated through verbal remarks and changes in the individual's behavior.

7. Nursing measures to assist patients in meeting psychological safety needs include:
   a. Pre-operative teaching
   b. Anxiety reduction techniques
   c. Assistance in developing effective coping strategies
   d. Assistance in developing effective problem-solving skills
   e. Assistance in coping with body image alterations
   f. Orientation to unfamiliar environments
   g. Explanations regarding treatment, tests and procedures

SECTION 4: Loving and Belonging Needs

A. Loving and belonging needs

1. Third-level needs involve feelings of loving and belonging.

2. People with well developed self-concepts generally need to feel loved and accepted by their families, peers, and other members of their community.

3. When individuals become ill, or suffer from injuries, they can find it difficult to meet these needs because of such health care delivery system issues as organization, environmental limitations, routines, and visiting hours.

4. Indicators that patients are not meeting loving and belonging needs may include:
   a. Changes in physical appearance, especially hygiene
   b. Isolation behavior
   c. Somatic complaints
   d. Verbal statements of loneliness
   e. Irritability
   f. Crying and acting out behaviors

5. Nursing measures to assist patients in meeting loving and belonging needs include:
   a. Creating opportunities for patients to have social interactions with family members and, when appropriate, other hospitalized individuals
   b. Maintaining social contacts through available resources
   c. Use of available community resources
   d. Encouraging patient participation in care planning

e. Providing the patient with access to spiritual care

SECTION 5: Self-Esteem Needs

A. Self-esteem needs

1. Fourth-level needs are those involving self-esteem, self-confidence, usefulness, achievement, and self worth.

2. An individual's self-esteem is linked to the desire for strength, achievement, adequacy, mastery, competence, independence, and freedom.

3. Common threats to a person's sense of self-esteem can include:
   a. Changes in roles, role strain, and role conflict
   b. Alteration in body image
   c. Significant actual or perceived losses
   d. Alteration in significant interpersonal relationships
   e. Loss of independence
   f. Inability to meet personal or professional goals and ambitions

4. Indicators that individuals have unmet self-esteem needs include:
   a. Negative statements about themselves
   b. Deferred decision-making and problem-solving
   c. Lethargy or apathy
   d. Feelings of hopelessness and helplessness
   e. Lack of motivation
   f. Lack of confidence
   g. Inability to find pleasure in life

5. Assisting patients to meet self-esteem needs, nursing measures focus on improving the patient's self-concept and body image.

SECTION 6: Self-Actualization Needs

A. Self-actualization needs

1. The last level of needs involves self-actualization, a state of fully achieving one's potential to solve problems and cope with life.

2. A self-actualized individual in Western cultures:

      a. Is autonomous and motivated
      b. Solves his or her own problems
      c. Accepts assistance from others
      d. Provides assistance to others
      e. Balances needs and stressors
      f. Is flexible in dealings with others
      f. Adapts to change and demands

3. How well the person can maintain a sense of self-actualization depends upon present need demands, environment, and exposure to stressors.

4. Illness, injury, or disease can cause frustration, self-centeredness, increased dependency on others, and decreased motivation.

5. Nursing measures to assist patients in meeting self-actualization needs focus on attaining or restoring a self-actualized state:
      a. Encouraging participation in decision-making
      b. Encouraging active involvement in planning and implementing care
      c. Providing opportunities for patient creativity
      d. Providing privacy
      e. Avoiding undue restriction on the patient's activities which promote autonomy, motivation, or independence

Unit 4

HOMEOSTASIS, ADAPTATION, HEALTH AND ILLNESS

C*hange and instability are essential for life. However, a degree of consistency and stability is fundamental in dealing with a stressful environment. To survive, individuals must satisfactorily adapt to change. Health is the ability to function fully and to find expression in all aspects of one's life. The eventual consequence of a state in which needs are continually unmet is system disequilibrium and, ultimately, illness. This unit presents basic concepts associated with homeostasis and adaptation to biological and psychological stressors. The effects of illness and hospitalization on the person are also addressed.*

SECTION 1: Homeostasis and Adaptation to Stress

A. Homeostasis

1. Homeostasis is an internal dynamic form of equilibrium.
2. Homeostasis is the body's tendency to maintain a state, or condition, of relative constancy.
3. Physiological mechanisms that maintain homeostasis.
   a. Homeostasis mechanisms are self-regulatory, functioning through a process of negative feedback, and compensating for abnormal states.
   b. Generally these mechanisms are controlled by the central nervous system (sympathetic and parasympathetic) and operate on an unconscious level.
   c. Three major homeostasis mechanism controls.
      - Medulla Oblongata – controls vital body functions, such as heart rate and respiratory rate, by increasing or decreasing their activity.
      - Reticular Formation – controls vital body functions and monitors physiological states of the body through both sensory and motor nerve tracts.
      - Pituitary Gland – supplies hormones that are necessary for:
        1. Adaptation to stresses
        2. Regulation of growth, thyroid, parathyroid, and gonadal hormone secretion
        3. Controlling vital system functions
4. Limitations to homeostasis control.
   a. Homeostasis mechanisms function together through complex relationships among the nervous system, hormonal levels, and body systems.
   b. These mechanisms can provide only short-term control over equilibrium.
   c. Long-term situations such as illness, injury, and disease can decrease the capacity for homeostasis.
   d. The feedback processes of homeostasis can also break down because of an abnormality within organs and/or systems.
   e. When limitations to homeostasis occur, health care professionals intervene to restore homeostasis.

B. Concepts of stress and adaptation

1. Stress and stressors.
   a. Stress is encountered by everyone in everyday living.

    b. Stress can be a positive experience, stimulating change and growth, or it can be a negative experience resulting in poor judgment, physical illness or the inability to cope with stressful events.

    c. The nature of stressors can vary greatly. They can be perceived as unpleasant events such as going to the dentist, or as positive events such as graduating from school.

    d. Stress affects the whole person and threatens a person's equilibrium by:
- Disrupting homeostasis
- Threatening emotional well-being
- Altering normal perceptions of reality, problem-solving ability, and cognitive function
- Threatening relationships with others
- Threatening one's outlook on life

    e. Stressors can be anything—an object, an event, person, or a situation—in either the internal or external environment that requires a response to decrease the stress.
- Internal stressors originate within the person.
- External stressors originate outside of the person.

2. Current models used to explain stress and the stress response.
    a. Psychosomatic Model
    b. Adaptation Model
    c. Social environment Model
    d. Process Model

3. Factors influencing the stress response.
    a. Responses to stressors will depend of the characteristics of the person and on the nature or the stressor.
    b. Personal variables influencing stress responses include:
- Personality
- Past stressful experiences
- Success or failure of past coping strategies.

    c. Characteristics of stressor variables which can influence one's response to stress include:
- Intensity of the stressor
- Scope of the stressor
- Duration of exposure to the stressor
- Number and nature of other stressors present.

4. Concept of adaptation.

    a. Adaptation is an attempt to maintain optimal levels of functioning.

    b. Human adaptation involves the use of:
- Reflexes
- Autonomic body mechanisms for protection
- Coping mechanisms
- Instincts

5. Dimensions of adaptation.

    a. Physical-developmental dimension
- Each developmental stage involves particular tasks and particular potential stressors. Each is characterized by certain adaptive responses to stress.
- Physiological adaptive responses are stimulated by stressors in either the internal or external environment.
- Physiological responses to stress may be limited to a specific body area (local adaptation) or the entire body (general adaptation).

    b. Affective dimension.
Each individual responds to stressors in his or her own manner. There are two types of psychological adaptive behaviors.
- Task-oriented behaviors (deliberate problem-solving methods)
  1. Asking questions
  2. Attack behavior
  3. Withdrawal behavior
  4. Compromise behavior

- Ego-defense mechanisms, conscious or unconscious mental processes.
  1. Suppression – conscious removal of unaccepted feelings and thoughts from awareness.
  2. Undoing – attempting to counteract the effects of doing something.
  3. Denial – refusal to accept or process unacceptable thoughts, feelings, wishes, needs, or events.
  4. Displacement – transferring emotions from their original source to one that is less threatening.
  5. Identification – patterning oneself after another person.
  6. Regression – unconscious elimination of unacceptable thoughts, events, or impulses.
  7. Projection – rejection of unacceptable feelings or thoughs by attributing them to others.

8.   Rationalization – justifying or making tolerable that which is actually intolerable.
   c. Intellectual dimension.
      A person's intellectual dimension includes:
      • Intellectual capacity and educational development
      • Perceptions of the world and other people
      • Communication patterns
      • Problem-solving and decision-making styles
      Intellectual adaptation is effected by emotions and can involve gathering information, solving problems, and communicating with others.

C. Psychophysiological response to stress

1.   Physiological component of the stress response.
   a. Local Adaptation Syndrome (LAS) is a response of tissue, organ, or body part to a stressor.
   b. Characteristics of a local adaptation response:
      • The response is localized and does not involve the entire body.
      • A stressor is necessary to stimulate the response.
      • The response is short-term
      • The response assists to restore homeostasis in some part of the body.

   c. Examples of two localized responses:
      • Reflex pain response - touching a hot pot handle
      • Inflammatory response - swelling at the site of an insect sting

   d. General Adaptation Syndrome (GAS) is a response of the whole body to stress.
      • A general adaptive response primarily involves the autonomic nervous system and the endocrine system (neuroendrocrine response).
      • Three stages of a general adaptation response are:
         1.   Alarm Reaction – body mobilizes mechanisms to adapt to a stressor
         2.   Resistance Stage – body stabilizes, vital functions return to normal, and adaptation continues
         3.   Exhaustion Stage – if stress cannot be resisted, energy to maintain adaptation is expended; the physiological response is intensified; adaptation to stressor lessens; and the body can no longer defend itself against the stressor.

D. The effects of prolonged exposure to stress

1. Strong correlation has been found between prolonged stress and cardiovascular illness, gastrointestinal illness, and cancer.

2. The intensity of a stressor, and the duration of exposure to the stress, appear to be variables crucial to influencing the onset, course, and recovery stages of illness.

3. Prolonged stress can interrupt or delay passage through developmental stages, or it may cause a maturational crisis.

4. Prolonged stress affects mental well-being and can result in mental illness.

5. A correlation has been found between intense, or prolonged, stress exposure and an increase in substance abuse.

6. Prolonged stress can reduce abilities to acquire new knowledge and skills, decrease communication effectiveness, and interfere with problem solving ability.

7. Prolonged stress can result in changes in normal behavioral patterns, role performance and expectations, and social interaction.

SECTION 2: Health and Illness

A. Defining health and illness

1. Defining the concept of health is very difficult.

2. Health is not merely the absence of illness; nor is it an acquired piece of knowledge, or a function of the body.

3. Health is a dynamic "state of being" defined by each person based upon his or her values and beliefs.

4. The World Health Organization (WHO) definition of health (1974):
   a. The WHO defined health as a state of complete physical, mental and social well-being, not merely the absence of disease or infirmity.
   b. Limitations to the WHO definition of health:
   - The definition is unrealistic for use with individuals living in underdeveloped countries or persons of low socioeconomic status who could never be considered healthy according to this definition

- Use of this definition makes it difficult to determine scientifically who is, or is not, healthy, nor the point at which one becomes ill or healthy.

5. Health and illness must be defined in terms of the individual. The patient's concept of health is very important to the nurse when assisting him or her to reach health care goals, which will also vary in each individual.

6. Since attitudes of clients and nurses toward health may not coincide, the nurse must work with the patient and family, to establish mutual goals of care and the plan of care.

   Example: Mexican-American migrant farm workers do not perceive themselves as being "sick" until they are no longer able to go out to work in the fields.

7. Acute illness refers to alterations in health states which have a severe, rapid onset of pronounced symptoms, and are usually of short duration.

   Example: Acute Appendicitis

8. Chronic illnesses are caused by irreversible pathologic alterations of the body which result in disabilities and the need for rehabilitation, long term medical supervision, and direct nursing care.

   Example: Chronic Obstructive Pulmonary Disease (COPD)

B. Current models of health and illness

1. A model is a theoretical way of understanding complex concepts.

2. Health models have been developed that can help nurses:
   a. Understand health behaviors and beliefs
   b. Predict health behaviors
   c. Predict the use of health services and adherence to recommended therapies
   d. Help the patient regain and maintain a high level of wellness
   e. Assess patient risk factors, illness patterns, life-style, physiological and behavioral functioning

3. Health beliefs are a person's ideas, convictions, and attitudes about health and illness that are based on factual information, misinformation, common sense, common myths, reality, or false expectations.

4. Health beliefs support activities called health behaviors that may positively or negatively affect health.

a. Positive health behaviors are related to maintaining, attaining, or regaining good health and preventing illness.

b. Negative health behaviors include practices that are potentially detrimental to health and well-being.

5. Health and illness models are approaches chosen to understand complex issues of patient attitudes and behavior toward health and illness. Health and disease models have shifted focus over time from superstition, to the individual, to wholeness, and, currently, to the relationship between individuals and their environment.

a. Health-Illness Continuum Model.
- Health and illness are relative qualities rather than absolute states.
- Health is seen as a dynamic state that changes continually as the person adapts to changes in internal and external environments to maintain a state of physical, emotional, intellectual, social, and spiritual wellness.
- Illness is an abnormal process which results in a diminished or impaired functioning.
- A patient's level of health can be located at any point on the continuum between high level wellness and severe illness.
- The client's view of his or her present level of health depends on attitudes toward health, values, beliefs, and perception of well-being.
- The nurse's role is to assist the patient in accurately identifying his or her position on the health/illness continuum.
- The Continuum Model is effective when used to compare the patient's present level of health with previous levels of health, and for setting goals for attaining a desired level of health.
- A limitation in the use of the Continuum Model is that it is not always easy to describe a client's level of health in terms of the two extremes.

b. Dunn's High-Level Wellness Model.
- Optimal health, or high-level wellness, is described as a state in which the person's functioning is balanced, purposeful, and directed toward attaining full potential.
- This is a holistic approach focusing on integrated well-being as the basis for health.
- Health care is directed toward assisting patients to achieve high-level wellness, emphasizing the

promotion of health promotion and the prevention of illness.
- This model is applicable for the individual, the family, and community health.

c. Agent-Host-Environment Model.
- The level of health or illness depends on the dynamic relationships and interactions among three variables.
    1. The agent – any factor, internal or external, that by its presence or absence can lead to disease or illness.
    2. The host – that which is susceptible to illness to disease.
    3. The environment – physical, social, economic, or other factors that increase the likelihood of experiencing disease or illness.
- The model seeks a source or cause of illness.

d. Health Beliefs Model.
- The Health Beliefs Model is characterized by the relationships between a person's beliefs and actions.
- This model addresses the role of:
    1. A person's perception of his susceptibility to illness
    2. A person's perception of the seriousness of the illness
    3. The psychological- and demographic-modifying factors affecting the probability of the person taking recommended actions. The probabilty is based upon one's perception of the benefits of the action.

e. Holistic Health Model.
- Holism is a theme from the humanities.
- This model provides an approach to health and health care that identifies and respects the interaction of mind, body, and spirit within an environment.
- Holism is based on the belief that the person cannot be understood when examined in parts or outside an environment.
- Holistic practice involves:
    1. Self-responsibility
    2. Informed choices
    3. Self-worth
    4. Meaning assigned to disease, illness, and dysfunction
    5. The effects of stress

C. Variables influencing health beliefs and practices

1. Internal variables influencing health beliefs and practices that must be assessed and considered when planning and implementing nursing care.
   a. Developmental stage and emotional development
   b. Intellectual background, past experiences, and cognitive abilities
   c. Perceptions of physical functioning level
   d. Emotional and spiritual factors

2. External Variables influencing health beliefs and practices that must be assessed and considered when planning and implementing nursing care.
   a. Family health practices and behaviors
   b. Use of availale health care services
   c. Social and psychological factors:
      • Economic factors
      • Stability of interpersonal relationships and social networks
      • Occupational environment
      • Life-style habits

   d. Cultural/Ethnic background factors:
      • Cultural values and customs
      • Cultural language
      • Cultural behaviors
      • Cultural perception of reality

D. Health promotion and illness prevention

1. Three levels of health activities are directed toward health promotion and illness prevention.
   a. Primary Level
      • Actions are taken to maintain and improve health and to prevent future illness
      • Focus is on general populations or particular identified, "at risk" groups not currently experiencing health problems.
         Examples: health education programs, immunization programs
   b. Secondary Level
      • Actions are taken to regain and/or restore functional level.
      • Focus is on individuals currently experiencing health problems or illness and who are at risk for developing complications

> > *Examples:* wound care, ambulating and range of
> > motion exercises, administering oxygen
> > therapy

  c. Tertiary Level
- Actions are taken to help patients adapt to limitations in functioning caused by illness, injury, or disease. Actions also are taken for preventing further disability.
- Focus is on individuals with disabilities both short-term and long term.

> > *Examples:* patient teaching regarding home safely
> > when oxygen is in use, infectious
> > disease contact follow-up

2. Risk Factors.
  a. Situations, habits, conditions, or other variables that increase vulnerability to injury or disease include:
- Genetic and physiological factors
- Age and developmental stage
- Environment
- Life-style and individual behavior

F. Illness and illness behavior

1. Variables influencing illness behavior can be categorized as internal or external.
  a. Internal variables affecting illness behavior include:
- Perceptions of symptoms and the degree of severity of the symptoms
- Nature of the illness, whether an acute episode or chronic illness
- Acute illness may result in:
  1. An increase in patient actions regarding the seeking of health care
  2. Active patient involvement in their care
  3. Increased adherence to the suggested therapeutic regimen
- Chronic illness can result in:
  1. Patient frustration
  2. Less active involvement in care and health decisions
  3. Reduced adherence to suggested therapeutic regimens.

  b. External variables affecting illness behavior include:
- Visibility of symptoms or recognition by others of the dysfunction
- Social network support systems
- Cultural background
- Economic variables

- Accessibility to health care systems

2. Five stages, or patterns, of illness behavior often experienced while seeking, finding, and interacting with the health care system have been identified. Progression through these stages will vary with the individual.

   a. Stage 1: Symptom experience
      - There is a perception that "something is wrong," but no specific diagnosis is suspected.
      - Perceptions include: an awareness of a physical change; an evaluation of the perceived change; and, if an illness is suspected, an emotional response.
      - Behavior following acknowledgment of a symptom can include any or all of the following:
         1. Self-medicating behavior
         2. Seeking immediate health care
         3. Denial of the symptom's presence or meaning
         4. Delay in seeking health care

   b. Stage 2: Assumption of the sick role
      - There is acknowledgment of the presence of a health problem.
      - The illness becomes a social phenomenon (known to others).
      - The person seeks confirmation from his or her family and social groups.
      - Normal roles and responsibilities are relinquished.
      - Both physical and emotional changes occur.
      - Behavior following acknowledgment of an illness requiring intervention can include any or all of the following:
         1. Continued use of lay remedies
         2. Denying required intervention
         3. Delaying contact with the health care system
         4. Care-seeking behavior

   c. Stage 3: Medical care contact
      - If the symptoms persist, become more severe, or require emergency attention, there is a motivation to seek professional care to obtain expert validation of illness and a course of treatment.
      - The individual also seeks an explanation for the symptoms, cause of symptoms, information about the course of the illness, and future implication of one's health state.
      - The person either accepts or rejects the professional diagnosis.

        1.   If the person accepts the diagnosis, he or she generally will follow through with the suggested course of treatment.

        2.   If the person rejects the diagnosis, he or she may begin to "shop around", consulting health care providers until one is found who makes a diagnosis desired by the person or the person accepts the original diagnosis.

  d. Stage 4: Dependency client role
- When the person accepts his or her illness, and seeks treatment, he or she becomes dependent on health care professionals for symptom relief and accepts care, sympathy, and protection from the demands and stressors of life.
- At this stage the person is given permission to be relieved of normal obligations and roles by society, and must adjust to disruption of his or her daily schedule.

  e. Stage 5: Recovery and rehabilitation
- Recovery and rehabilitation may occur abruptly or over a long period of time.
- In the case of chronic illness this stage may be a prolonged period of adjustment to reduce functioning and altered state of health.

G. Summary of the impaired role versus sick role

1. The impaired role.
   a. Role expectations for the impaired person tend to be more supportive of normal behavior.
   b. The impaired person is encouraged to be independent in personal care and social responsibilities.
   c. The impaired person is encouraged to seek appropriate medical care.
   d. The impaired person does not expect to be given complete information regarding his or her health state.
   e. The impaired person is not insulated from family and work responsibilities or concerns.
   f. The impaired person is rarely isolated from the well population.
2. The sick role.
   a. Those considered sick are thought to have disorders that are more serious, incapacitating, and life-threatening.
   b. The sick person is expected to be dependent on others for care.
   c. The sick person is entitled to a great deal of extra care.

    d. The sick person is insulated from family and personal responsibilities, difficulties, and concerns.

    e. The sick person requires complete information regarding their health status.

    f. The sick person is isolated from the well population.

H. Impact of illness on patients and family

1. Illness is not experienced as an isolated event. Families and social networks must adjust to changes resulting from illness, injury, disease, and treatment of the "identified" patient.

2. Possible emotional responses by the person, family or community to illness, injury, disease, or hospitalization.

    a. Anxiety – a sense of apprehension, unease, or uncertainty that occurs in anticipation of some threat.

    b. Shock – an adaptive emotional state, described as being "numb" or "immobilized", that allows individuals to absorb threatening events or information.

    c. Denial – a mental defense mechanism that allows individuals to avoid emotional conflict and anxiety, refusing to acknowledge facts that are intolerable. Denial can be a very effective way of coping as long as it does not interfere with treatment or therapy.

    d. Anger – an emotional response that may take rational or irrational forms, directed through a variety of outlets and toward a variety of receptors.

    e. Withdrawal – often a symptom of depression or a response to anger involving isolation, avoiding interaction with others.

3. Possible behavioral responses to illness, injury, disease, or hospitalization.

    a. Fearfulness

    b. Regressive behavior

    c. Egocentric behavior, preoccupation with the self

    d. Emotional overreaction

    e. Over-emphasis of insignificant concerns (Blow-up behavior)

    f. Altered perception of others

4. Impact of illness on self-concept.

    a. Self-concept is a mental image of oneself.

    b. Changes in self-concept may be more complex and less easily observable than changes in roles or body image.

    c. Self-concept is very important to the patient's relationships with family and social networks.

5. Impact of illness on body image.
    a. Body image is a subconcept of physical appearance.
    b. A patients reaction to a change in his or her physical appearance and body image often depend upon:
- Type of change involved
- Visibility of the change
- Adaptive capacity of the person and/or family members
- Rate at which the change takes place
- The supportive services available to the person and/or family

6. People generally respond to a change in body image in four phases:
    a. Impact (shock) – depersonalization of the experience by the patient. Nursing actions are directed toward:
- Providing emotional and physical support
- Making no demands on the patient nor forcing decision-making
- Providing truthful answers to patient questions
- Offering brief explanations

    b. Retreat (withdrawal) – both patient and family experiencing an increase in anxiety may withdraw and flee. Nursing interventions are directed toward:
- Providing emotional and physical support
- Not forcing reality until patient is ready
- Helping patient accept reality in small increments
- Re-organizing inner resources to prepare to move ahead

    c. Acknowledgment – as the patient mourns the losses, others must change their concept of the patient. The patient may be argumentative, sarcastic, suicidal. Nursing interventions are directed toward:
- Continuously assessing level of depression
- Providing emotional and physical support
- Exploring the meaning of the change for the patient
- Assisting patient to direct anger in positive directions
- Encouraging the patient to have contact with the changed body part (visual, tactile)
- Identifying how the change will affect various aspects of the patient's life
- Aleviating feeling of shame or stigma
- Encouraging and stressing independence

    d. Restructuring (rehabilitation) – adjustment to technical devices and procedures. The patient reorganizes social values and reintegrates his or her self-image. Nursing interventions are directed toward:
- Identifying meanings of multiple changes for the patient
- Identifying the impact of changes upon people with whom the patient interacts.
- Identifying the significance of the physical changes for significant others
- Identifing alterations in work roles and recreational activities
- Encouraging the sharing of the experience with others

7. Impact of illness on family role, task expectations, and accomplishment.
    a. The patient's various role within the family must be identified.
    b. A role change in one person always results in role changes for others who interact with that person.
    c. Role changes may be subtle and short-term, or drastic and long-term.
    d. Short-term role changes usually do not require prolonged adjustment periods, but long-term role changes may require an adjustment phase similar to the grieving process.
    e. Although an ill person needs the opportunity to recover following a change in health state, this does imply that they must relinquish all family roles and responsibilities.

8. Impact of illness on family dynamics.
    a. "Family dynamics" refers to the process by which the family functions as a whole, makes decisions, provides support, and copes with changes and challenges.
    b. A shift to a new pattern of family functioning is often the result of illness, especially prolonged illness; this shift can create severe stress for family members.

Unit 5

BASIC SKILLS FOR
BEGINNING LEVEL ASSESSMENT

A*ssessment data forms the foundation of the nursing process. A comprehensive, accurate data base is critical for designing a plan of patient care and for evaluating the effectiveness of nursing interventions. Performing physical and psychological assessment is a challenging aspect of nursing care. Performing health assessment is a primary nursing responsibility in hospitals, clinics, physicians' offices, at health fairs, and at home. This unit provides a general summary of assessment. Information in this unit will assist in developing beginning level physical assessment and psychological assessment skills. It also will assist in understanding the nurse's role in diagnostic tests and procedures. It is impossible to develop accurate assessment skills without supervised practice. An understanding of normal human physical structure and function and human psychology is prerequisite to assessment skill development.*

SECTION 1: Basic Beginning Physical Assessment

A. The physical examination

1. The purposes of physical examinations are:
   a. Routine screening
   b. Eligibility for employment, school activities, physical activities, medical insurance, military service
   c. Hospital admission
   d. Establishing a data base for the patient
   e. Identifying patient problems requiring intervention
   f. Evaluating the effectiveness of care
   g. Developing credibility for promoting the nurse/patient relationship

2. Nurses in all health care settings typically perform complete physical examinations.

3. In all settings the physical examination should be integrated into the nurse's routine care.

4. The nurse must first learn to identify normal characteristics before attempting to distinguish abnormal findings.

B. Techniques necessary for an accurate physical examination

1. Observation and measurement.

2. Inspection – visual and olfactory inspection to observe color, odor, size, shape, symmetry, and movement.

3. Palpation – using the sense of touch simultaneously with inspection to identify softness, rigidity, temperature, and to determine position, size, texture, consistency, and moisture

4. Auscultation – listening to sounds (usually with stethoscope) produced by their frequency, intensity, quality, and duration. Low pitched sounds are better heard with the bell of the stethoscope, and high pitched sounds are heard better with the stethoscope's diaphragm.

5. Percussion – striking body surfaces, producing sounds to determine if underlying tissues are air-filled, fluid-filled, or solid.
   Percussion sounds include:
   - Flat (non resonant; soft tissues)
   - Dull (thudlike; solid organs)
   - Resonant (hollow)
   - Hyperresonant (booming)
   - Tympanic (over gas-filled organs; drumlike)

C. Preparation for the examination

1. The environment must be suitable and all equipment gathered before examination begins.
2. Preparation of the environment.
    a. The examination is performed in privacy.
    b. Adequate lighting is required for proper illumination of body parts, observation, and inspection.
    c. The examination room should be soundproof if possible; if not, all extraneous noise should be eliminated.
    d. The examination table should feel comfortable to the patient.
3. Preparation of the equipment.
    a. Equipment and hands should be kept warm.
    b. All equipment should function properly.
    c. All equipment should be gathered prior to the beginning of the examination and should be kept within easy reach of the examiner.
4. Physical preparation of the patient.
    a. The patient should be asked to void prior to the examination.
    b. The reason for specimen collection as well as procedures for their collection should be explained to the patient.
    c. The patient should be properly positioned and draped for examination.
    d. The patient should be keep warm and out of drafts; seriously ill patients are more susceptible to chills.
    e. The patient should be provided with privacy and adequate time to dress and undress.
5. Psychological preparation of the patient.
    a. Provide reassurance and support to decrease patient anxiety and embarrassment.
    b. Explain actions clearly and in detail using simple explanations.
    c. Acquire a third person to be in the examination room when the patient and examiner are of the opposite sex.
    d. Monitor the patient's emotional responses throughout the examination.

D. Positioning for physical examination

1. Sitting.

    a. Sitting upright provides good visualization of the symmetry of the upper body and allows full expansion of the lungs.

    b. Areas assessed with the patient in a sitting position include:
- Head and neck
- Thorax and lungs
- Breasts
- Axilla
- Heart
- Vital signs
- Upper extremities

    c. Physically weak patients may not be able to sit. A supine position with the head of the bed elevated can be used instead.

2. Supine.

    a. The supine position is normally the most relaxed position; it prevents contracture of abdominal muscles and provides easy access to pulse points.

    b. Areas assessed with the patient in the supine position include:
- Head and neck
- Anterior thorax and lungs
- Axilla
- Heart
- Abdomen
- Extremities
- Pulse points

    c. The supine position may be difficult for patients experiencing shortness of breath.

3. Dorsal recumbent.

    a. Bending the knees in the dorsal recumbent position may be more comfortable for patients with painful disorders.

    b. Areas assessed with the patient in the dorsal recumbent position include:
- Head and neck
- Anterior thorax and lungs
- Breasts
- Axilla
- Heart

    c. This position cannot be used to assess the abdomen since it promotes contracture of the abdominal muscles.

4. Lithotomy.

      a. The Lithotomy position provides the greatest exposure of genitalia and allows insertion of the vaginal speculum.

      b. The female genitalia is assessed with the patient in the lithotomy position.

      c. Severe arthritis or other joint deformities may prevent patients from assuming this position.

5. Sims'.

      a. The patient in the prone position with the hips and knees flexed provides exposure of the rectal area.

      b. The rectum is assessed with the patient in the Sims' position.

      c. Joint deformities may prevent the patients from assuming this position.

E. Sequence for a general survey

1. Assess vital signs.

      a. Pulse (rate, rhythm, quality)

      b. Respiration (rate, depth, pattern, effort)

      c. Temperature

      d. Blood pressure (sitting, standing)

2. Measure height and weight.

3. Assess general appearance.

      a. Age

      b. Race

      c. Sex

      d. Body type

      e. Posture

      f. Gait

      g. General body build

      h. Coordination

4. Integument.

      a. Assessment of the entire skin surface can be performed at once, or each body area can be assessed separately.

      b. Assessment of integument requires skills of inspection, palpation, and olfaction.

      c. Characteristics assessed include:

          • Color (cyanosis, jaundice, pallor)

          • Temperature

          • Texture

          • Turgor and mobility

          • Lesions and rashes

          • Vascularity (petechiae, ecchymosis, edema)

          • Odors

5. Head and neck.
   a. Hair
      - Observe hair distribution, thickness, texture, and lubrication.
      - Palpate the scalp for lesions.
      - Inspect the hair for head lice or other vermin.

   b. Head
      - Inspect the head, noting size, shape, and contour.
      - Palpate the temporal pulse point (rate, rhythm, strength, quality of pulses).

   c. Neck
      - Palpate and auscultate the carotid arteries.
      - Inspect the neck, noting symmetry, edema, masses, scars.
      - Palpate lymph nodes, noting size, tenderness.
      - Inspect and palpate the thyroid gland, noting enlargement, masses, nodules.
      - Palpate the trachea, noting alignment, masses.
      - Inspect jugular veins, noting distention.
      - Assess range of motion, noting limitations, pain.
      - Assess sternocleidomastoid strength.
      - Assess spinal accessory nerve function (head shoulder movement).

   d. Face
      - Inspect face, noting size, shape, symmetry, tics.
      - Assess facial nerve function (facial expression).

   e. Eyes (inflammation, lesions, edema, pitosis)
      - Assess optic nerve function (visual acuity).
      - Assess visual fields.
      - Assess Extraoccular movements.
      - Assess abducens nerve function (lateral eyeball movement).
      - Assess trigeminal nerve function (upward/downward eyeball movement).
      - Assess occulomoter nerve function (pupil constriction and dilatation).
      - Assess external structures (alignment, eyebrows, eyelids, lacrimal apparatus, conjunctivae and sclerae, pupils and iris).

   f. Nose
      - Inspect the nose noting symmetry, inflammation, deformity, discoloration, edema, discharge, swelling, epitaxis, obstruction.

- Inspect nasal mucosa and septum (color, symmetry, swelling, bleeding).
- Palpate the frontal and maxillary facial area for tenderness.
- Assess olfactory nerve function (sense of smell).

g. Ears
  - Inspect the condition of the outer and middle ear structures (inflammation, foreign bodies, pain, discharge).
  - Palpate the external structures.
  - Assess auditory acuity (location of sound, air and bone conduction).
  - Assess for mechanical dysfunction, neurological disorders, trauma, acute illness.
  - Inquire about pain, itching, discharge, tinnitus, or hearing change.

h. Mouth and pharynx
  - Evaluate quality of oral hygiene.
  - Inspect lips, noting color, texture, hydration, contour, lesions, symmetry.
  - Inspect oral mucosa noting color, hydration, texture, ulcers, abrasions, cysts.
  - Inspect gums or gingivae noting color, edema, retraction, bleeding, lesions, inflammation.
  - Inspect teeth noting alignment, caries, extraction, teeth color.
  - Inspect the tongue on all sides for color, size, texture, position in the mouth, lesions, mobility.
  - Assess hypoglossal nerve function (position of tongue).
  - Inspect the palate noting color, shape, defects.
  - Inspect the uvula and soft palate, noting edema, color, petechiae, lesions.
  - Assess jaw range of motion, noting limitations, pain.
  - Assess glossopharyngeal nerve function (taste).
  - Assess vagus nerve function (swallowing).

6. Arms, hands, and fingers.
   a. Inspect nails for color, thickness, shape, and curvature.
   b. Palpate the nails to assess circulation or capillary filling (blanching).
   c. Palpate the brachial and radial arteries (rate, rhythm, strength, quality of pulses).
   d. Assess range of motion of all joints noting limitation, pain.
      - Shoulder
      - Elbow

- Wrist
- Fingers

e. Assess muscle strength.
- Trapezius
- Biceps
- Triceps

f. Assess grip strength in both hands.

g. Assess motor function.
- Coordination
- Balance

h. Assess sensory function, noting sensation of pain, touch, position, vibration, two point discrimination.

7. Thorax and lungs.
   a. Posterior thorax
   - Inspect the chest, noting shape, deformities, position of the spine, slope of the ribs, retraction or bulging of intercostal spaces.
   - Inspect the scapulae, noting symmetry.
   - Palpate the chest, noting lumps, masses, tenderness.
   - Measure exertion and elicit tactile fremitus.
   - Systematically percuss chest wall, noting resonance.
   - Systematically auscultate breath sounds, noting adventitious or abnormal sounds (crackles, rales, wheezes, ronchi).

   b. Lateral thorax
   - With the patient's arms extended straight up in the air, extend posterior thorax assessment.

   c. Anterior thorax
   - Inspect for the same features observed in the posterior thorax assessment.
   - Palpate for areas, noting abnormalities, tenderness, excursion, tactile fremiyus.
   - Systematically percuss the anterior chest.
   - Systematically auscultate the anterior chest.

8. Heart.
   a. Assess apical pulse (rate, rhythm, strength),
   b. Palpate the point of maximum impact (PMI).
   c. Auscultate the heart, noting abnormal sounds, extra sound, murmurs, arrhythmia
   - Aortic area S_2 loudest
   - Pulmonary area S_2 louder than S_1
   - Apical S_2 softer than S_1

9. Breasts.

    a. Inspect the breasts, noting size, shape, symmetry, contour.

    b. Inspect the skin, noting color, venous pattern, edema, inflammation.

    c. Inspect and palpate the nipples and areola, noting color, contour, symmetry, lesions, discharge.

    d. Palpate the breasts and lymph nodes, noting enlargement, tenderness, masses, consistency of breast tissue.

10. Abdomen.

    a. Inspect the skin surface, noting scars, venous pattern, lesions, striae, artificial openings, shape, symmetry, visible masses, movement.

    b. Inspect the umbilicus, noting position, shape, color, discharge, protruding mass.

    c. Systematically auscultate bowel sounds in all four quadrants, noting level of activity, normal, absent, hyperactive, or hypoactive sounds.

    d. Systematically percuss the abdomen, noting resonance, liver borders.

    e. Percuss each costovertebral angle at the scapular line, noting complaints of tenderness.

    f. Percuss the abdomen, noting to presence of ascites.

    g. Measure abdominal girth if ascites is suspected.

    h. Systematically palpate the abdomen, noting distention, masses, rebound tenderness, liver edge.

    i. Palpate the femoral arteries (rate, rhythm, strength, quality of pulses).

11. Legs, feet, and toes.

    a. Palpate the popliteal artery, posterior tibialis artery, and dorsalis pedis (rate, rhythm, strength, quality of pulses).

    b. Assess range of motion in all joints, noting limitation, pain.
- Hip
- Knee
- Ankle
- Toes

    c. Assess muscle strength.
- Quadriceps
- Gastrocnemius

    d. Assess Homan's sign, noting calf pain or soreness.

    e. Palpate for edema

    f. Inspect nails for color, thickness, shape, and curvature

g. Palpate the nails to assess circulation or capillary fill (blanching).

h. Assess motor function.
   • Coordination
   • Balance

i. Assess sensory function, noting sensation of pain, touch, position, vibration, two-point discrimination.

12. Common reflexes.

a. Reflexes are graded on a scale:
   • 0   no response
   • 1+ low-normal or abnormal
   • 2+ normal
   • 3+ brisker than normal
   • 4+ hyperactive, very brisk

b. Biceps – flexion of arm at elbow, noting grading of response.

c. Triceps – extension at elbow, noting grading of response.

d. Patellar – extension of lower leg at knee, noting grading of response.

e. Babinski (plantar) – flexion of toes, noting grading of response.

f. Achilles (ankle) – plantar flexion, noting grading of response.

F. Basic data gathering guide (Human needs approach)

1. Circulatory.

a. Blood Pressure

b. Pulses:
   • Carotid
   • Radial
   • Apical
   • Pedal
   • Rhythm

c. Skin/mucus membranes

d. Nail beds (color, blanching)

e. Skin temperature

f. I.V. placement

g. Diagnostic/lab data

h. Medications

2. Environmental.

a. Bed position

b. Side rails

      c. Restraints
      d. Equipment

3. Gastrointestinal.
      a. Diet
      b. Height and weight
      c. Amount ingested
      d. Bowel function (pattern, last bowel movement, bowel sounds)
      e. Abnormalities
      f. Medication
      g. Diagnostic/lab data
      h. Medications

4. Genito-urinary.
      a. Gender
      b. Significant other
      c. Concerns expressed
      d. Urination (pattern, appearance, amount)
      e. Urinary control
      f. Urinalysis results
      g. Medications
      h. Menses

5. Integumentary.
      a. Skin color
      b. Skin turgor
      c. Skin moisture
      d. Skin texture
      e. Lesions, wounds, scars, rashes
      f. Pressure areas
      g. Medications

6. Musculoskeletal.
      a. Posture
      b. Ability to move
      c. Joint range of motion
      d. Body alignment
      e. Activity tolerance
      f. Activity level ordered
      h. Rest periods
      i. Abnormalities
      j. Diagnostic/lab data
      k. Medications

7. Neural.

a. Speech
b. Vision
c. Hearing
d. Olfactory sense
d. Tactile sense
e. Sleep pattern
f. Gait
g. Pain:
  • Location
  • Duration
  • Cause
  • Intensity
  • Description

h. Diagnostic/lab data
i. Medications

8. Psychosocial.
  a. Age
  b. Life/developmental stage
  c. Occupation
  d. Position in family unit
  e. Hobbies and interests
  f. Religious/spiritual beliefs
  g. Support relationships
  h. Financial resources
  i. Emotional state:
    • Behaviors
    • Coping strategies
    • Mental defenses

  j. Communication style and barriers
  k. Self-concept

9. Respiratory.
  a. Respiration:
    • Rate
    • Rhythm
    • Depth
    • Chest movement

  b. Breath sounds
  c. Secretions
  d. Diagnostic/lab data
  e. Medications

G. Post examination

1. Clean any body areas examined where lubricants were used and clean any body secretions present.
2. After the examination is complete remove drapes and assist the patient with dressing.
3. Be certain that the patient is safe and comfortable.
4. Appropriately dispose of linens, pads, or equipment used.
5. Document examination findings using appropriate agency forms.
   a. History
   b. Physical assessment
   c. Psychosocial assessment
   d. Time of examination
   e. Name of examiner(s)
   f. Specimens collected and their disposition
   g. How the patient tolerated the examination process
   h. How and where the patient was left after the examination

SECTION 2: Beginning Level Psychosocial Assessment

A. Purpose of the psychosocial assessment

1. The psychosocial dimension of the person includes his or her mental and emotional, social, cultural/ethnic, and spiritual aspects.
2. The psychosocial assessment differs from the traditional medical-surgical history; the purpose of the psychosocial assessment is to see the uniqueness of the individual's personality.
3. Another purpose of the psychosocial assessment is to create a data base for identifying, monitoring, and evaluating human responses and problems.
4. The psychosocial assessment also provides an opportunity to create a data base for making judgments about the patient's health.
5. The mental status component of the psychosocial assessment helps to assess the patient's ability to understand what is happening to them and to determine the degree of cooperation with the care plan that may be expected from the patient.

B. Components of the psychosocial assessment

1. Communication skills are essential for conducting a complete and accurate psychosocial assessment.

2. Early establishment of rapport between patient and nurse during the initial interview will facilitate effective assessment.

3. The psychosocial assessment is composed of two parts: the psychosocial history, and the mental status examination.

4. When conducting the psychosocial history, the proper sequence is to ask questions and then listen to what the patient says and how he or she says it.

5. The purpose of conducting a mental status examination is to observe the patient's appearance, behavior, and communication, and to assess cognitive functioning.

C. The psychosocial history

1. Each health care agency provides a format for collecting and documenting the information obtained in the interview.

2. The interview should contain information regarding:
   a. Demographic or identifying information
   b. Presenting problem
   c. Medical/surgical history
   d. History of psychological health problems
   e. Family history
   f. Cultural/ethnic background information
   g. Military history
   h. Educational and vocational history
   i. Legal history
   j. Coping mechanisms
   k. Values, beliefs, and goals
   l. Current life status and style

D. The mental status examination

1. The mental status examination provides the opportunity to observe the patient's behaviors and responses as he or she interact during the assessment.

2. The mental status format will vary among agencies.

3. A complete mental status examination will consist of observations regarding:
   a. General appearance
      • Grooming (neat, clean, unkempt)
      • Comparison of stated age and apparent age

- General state of health (excellent, good, fair, poor)
- Appropriateness of dress and use of cosmetics
- Level of consciousness (alert, lethargic, confused, other)
- Manner of dress (street clothes, hospital gown; appropriate, bizarre)
- Posture (rigid, relaxed)
- Facial expression
- Distinct physical features

b. Behavior
- Relationship with interviewer (appropriate, indifferent, distant, defensive)
- Degree of activity (calm, restless, slowed)
- Eye contact (good, fair, poor)
- Movements (purposeful, without purpose)
- Gestures or mannerisms
- Repetitive actions

c. Communication
- Tone of voice
- Volume of speech
- Rate of speech
- Choice of words
- Unusual speech pattern
- Monotonous speech
- Ability to articulate ideas

d. Mood, or the pervasive, sustained emotion or overall climate that cannot be observed.
- Dysphoria
- Euphoria
- Lability
- Depressed
- Anxious
- Hostile
- Angry
- Elated

e. Affect, or the extreme expression of emotion that can be inferred by observing the patient.
- Appropriate
- Blunted affect
- Flat affect
- Vacant stare
- Sad
- Tense

    f. Cognitive functioning, or orientation
- Time
- Place
- Person
- Purpose

    g. Cognitive functioning, or memory
- Recent memory
- Remote memory

    h. Cognitive function, or intellectual functioning
- General level of intellectual function

    i. Cognitive functioning, or thinking
- Thought content
- Ability for abstract thinking
- Ability to reason logically
- Concrete thinking
- Ability to concentrate
- Thought processes, flow of ideas
- Preoccupation, obsessions
- Presence of illusions
- Presence of hallucinations
- Presence of delusions
- Judgment
- Insight

SECTION 3: Assessing Vital Signs

A. Rationale for the assessment of vital signs

1. Pulse, respiration, and temperature are components of basic assessment.

2. The professional nurse knows how to perform these basic measurement skills. He or she also understands the deviations from normal on which assessment and interpretations are based.

3. Temperature, pulse, and respiration are important indicators of a patient's physical status.

4. Vital signs are assessed:
   a. During a basic physical examination
   b. On admission
   c. As part of daily routine during hospitalization
   d. Before and after surgery or invasive diagnostic procedures

   e. When certain medications to control cardiac, respiratory, or temperature status are administered

   f. When patient's perceptions of his or her health state change

B. Body temperature

1. Body temperature indicates the balance between heat produced by the body and heat lost by the body.

2. An oral temperature reading of 98.6° F or 37° C. is generally a consistent finding in healthy, adult individuals.

3. Factors influencing body temperature include:
   a. Time of day
   b. Age
   c. Presence of infection
   d. Environmental temperature
   e. Metabolism
      • Muscular activity
      • Stimulation of sympathetic nervous system
      • Increased level of thyroxin
      • Oxidation of food
      • Fever
   f. Emotional status
   g. Hormones
   h. Ingestion of hot or cold foods or liquids (when temperature is taken orally)

4. Under normal conditions body heat is eliminated through four methods:
   a. Radiation
   b. Conduction
   c. Convection
   d. Evaporation

5. If temperature is elevated above normal, the patient is febrile.

6. Sites for measuring temperature include:
   a. Oral
   b. Rectal
   c. Axillary

7. Assessment of temperature is a simple measurement and each agency will have selected the equipment and established the procedures for measuring body temperature.

C. Pulse

1. Pulse rates vary greatly among adults. A pulse rate of 50 to 100 beats per minute is generally considered normal.

2. Factors influencing pulse rate include:
   a. Body temperature
   b. Exercise
   c. Application of hot and cold
   d. Medications
   e. Hemorrhage
   f. Heart disease
   g. Emotions
   h. Pain
   i. Stimulation of the vagus nerve
   j. Increased intracranial pressure

3. Pulse rates below 60 beats per minute are considered bradycardia.

4. Pulse rates above 100 beats per minute are considered tachycardia.

5. Pulses are measured by palpation at appropriate sites. The most common sites include:
   a. Temporal artery
   b. Carotid artery
   c. Radial artery
   d. Femoral artery
   e. Popliteal artery
   f. Posterior tibalis artery
   g. Dorsalis pedis artery

6. Pulses are described as:
   a. Regular
   b. Irregular
   c. Bounding
   d. Thready
   e. Weak
   f. Absent

7. The apical rate is measured by auscultation with the stethoscope.

8. Pulse rates can also be measured through the use of an ultrasound (Doppler) stethoscope.

9. A pulse deficit, a lower radial rate than the apical rate, when both are measured simultaneously, means that some of the

heart contractions are not strong enough to push a wave of blood sufficiently to be felt at the radial site.

10. Pulse rate, rhythm, and quality should be documented.

D. Respiration

1. Respiration is the act of breathing, an exchange of oxygen and carbon dioxide in the lungs and tissues.

2. Respiration involves inhalation and exhalation.

3. Respiration is an automatic and involuntary process mediated by the respiratory center located in the pons and medulla.

4. Normal respiration is described as effortless, automatic, regular, and even.

5. Types of noisy respiration include:
   a. Stridor – harsh inspiration, crowing sounds occurring with upper airway or laryngeal obstruction
   b. Wheeze – high-pitched musical whistling sounds occurring with partial obstruction in the bronchi and bronchioles
   c. Rhonchi – continuous course sounds caused by obstruction in the lager bronchi
   d. Sigh – deep inspiration.

6. Normal adults breathe 16 to 20 times per minute.

7. Respiratory disorders can significantly alter a person's respiratory pattern.

8. Difficulty in breathing is referred to as dsypnea.

9. Factors influencing respiratory rate include:
   a. Body temperature
   b. Exercise
   c. Application of hot and cold
   d. Medications
   e. Hemorrhage
   f. Heart disease
   g. Emotions
   h. Pain

10. Respiratory rate, depth, pattern, effort, and noise associated with breathing should be documented.

11. Four frequently encountered abnormal breathing patterns include:
    a. Cheyne-Stokes respiration
    b. Boit's respiration
    c. Kussmaul's respiration

      d. Apneustic respiration

E. Blood pressure

1. Blood pressure is the pressure exerted by the blood in the arteries of the body and is an indicator of the patient's circulatory status.

2. Adult blood pressure varies greatly, and a reading of 110/140 to 60/90 is generally considered normal.

3. A systolic pressure (point at which the heart is beating) over 160, or a diastolic pressure (point at which the heart is relaxing and filling with blood) over 100, is referred to as hypertension.

4. A systolic pressure below 100 is referred to as hypotension.

5. Factors influencing blood pressure include:
   a. Activity
   b. Anxiety
   c. Strong emotion
   d. Recent ingestion of food
   e. Disease
   f. Pain
   g. Personal characteristics
      • Age
      • Weight
      • Height
      • Race
      • Diet
      • Gender

6. A drop in blood pressure can result from any factor that causes blood vessels to dilate.

7. Postural or orthostatic hypotension is a sudden drop in blood pressure caused by a change in position.

8. Sources of error in assessing blood pressure:
   a. Falsely high readings
      • Use of inappropriate cuff size
      • Wrapping cuff too loosely or unevenly on the arm
      • Taking a reading after the patient eats a meal, while the patient is smoking, or when the patient has a distended bladder
      • Deflating the cuff too slowly

   b. Falsely low readings
      • Positioning arm about the level of the heart
      • Diminished hearing acuity

- Use of an inappropriate stethoscope

c. Falsely high or low readings
  - Defective manometer
  - Inaccurately calibrated manometer
  - Performing procedure incorrectly or while being distracted

SECTION 4: Assisting With Diagnostic Tests/Procedures

A. Nursing responsibilities regarding medical diagnostic procedures

1. Laboratory and diagnostic testing remain an important part of establishing a diagnosis.

2. Laboratory and diagnostic tests include procedures that can involve any part of the body or any body system.

3. It is essential for the nurse to be aware of:
   a. The purpose of an ordered test or procedure
   b. How to prepare the patient for various procedures or tests
   c. How the tests or procedures are performed
   d. Care requirements following tests or procedures

4. Diagnostic tests use special equipment to visualize or evaluate normal body functions.

5. Laboratory tests require the collection of specimens from patients which are tested and can identify abnormalities in functioning.

6. The role of the nurse in facilitating diagnostic and laboratory testing includes:
   a. Preparing the patient for tests and procedures
   b. Obtaining samples
   c. Supporting the patient during test and procedures
   d. Performing post procedure assessments
   e. Sharing the results of procedures and tests with member of the health care team.

7. Patient information obtained from laboratory testing and diagnostic procedures aids in:
   a. Assessing function
   b. Identifying dysfunction
   c. Identifying patients at risk for dysfunction
   d. The individualization of patient care

8. Nursing responsibilities include:
    a. Scheduling procedures or tests
    b. Instucting the patient prior to, during, and following the test or procedure
    c. Witnessing signatures for informed consent
    d. Physically preparating the patient
    e. Obtaining necessary supplies and equipment

B. Preparing the patient for diagnostic procedures

1. The nurse plays a major role in preparing the patient for diagnostic procedures and laboratory testing.
2. Nursing assessment prior to a diagnostic procedure includes:
    a. A review of the patient's history of drug or food allergies
    b. Assessment of the patient's knowledge of the procedure
    c. Assessment of the patient's ability to follow instructions and directions
    d. Assessment of the patient's ability to tolerate the procedure
    e. Assessment of baseline vital signs
3. All tests involving the same specimens or similar procedures should be performed at the same time.
4. When scheduling tests for the elderly or severely ill patient, or for patients with chronic health problems, care should be taken not to over-tire the patient with too many tests or procedures over a short time period.
5. Tests requiring fasting should be scheduled for the morning hours.
6. Tests should be ordered in proper collection sequence to ensure optimal results.
7. Patient teaching regarding tests and procedures can significantly relieve patient anxiety, encourage cooperation, and help the patient cope with painful procedures.
8. The patient's dietary or fluid restrictions should be monitored.
9. Physician's orders regarding routine medication administration prior to, and following, procedures and tests should be verified.
10. Be sure that all jewelry, hairpins, and clothing with metal fastening are removed prior to magnetic resonance imaging (MRI).

C. Providing care and support during diagnostic procedures

1. During tests and procedures, the nurse may be asked to:
   a. Set up equipment
   b. Provide equipment and specimen collection containers as they are required
   c. Label specimens
   d. Administer medications
   e. Provide for patient safely
   f. Provide documentation of the test or procedure

2. During procedures the nurse should monitor the patient for changes in:
   a. Vital signs
   b. Affect upon the patient
   c. Skin color
   d. Mental status

3. During procedures the nurse is often responsible for positioning the patient.
   a. Prone
   b. Supine
   c. Fowler's
   d. Dorsal recumbent
   e. Lithotomy
   f. Knee-chest position
   g. Trendelenburg's
   h. Left-side lying
   i. Sims'

4. The patient should never be left unattended on an examination table.

5. Providing patient support is a major role of the nurse during tests and procedures.

6. Universal precautions should be used for all tests involving collection of body fluids and all invasive procedures.

7. Blood should not be drawn from an extremity in which intravenous solutions or blood are infusing.

D. Providing post procedural care and comfort

1. Following the procedure, baseline data should be compared to current data.

2. Assessment following many procedures will be described in agency policies and procedures.

3. The nurse should be aware of possible post-procedure complications the patient might experience.

4. Pressure should be applied over all sites of venipuncture, and the area should be elevated if bleeding continues.

5. After angiographic examination, peripheral pulses distal to the catheter puncture site should be monitored and compared to the temperature and skin color of the involved extremities.

6. The patient should be encouraged to drink fluids after procedures involving contrast dyes unless contraindicated by the patient's health.

7. The patient's psychological and physical responses to procedures and tests should be comprehensively documented.

8. Cleaning the work area after a procedure may be the nurse's responsibility. Sharp objects and needles should be discarded in appropriate containers.

E. Laboratory tests

1. Protocols for sample collection provide information regarding the amount of specimen material to be collected and how specimens should be handled during transport and storage.

2. The patient's record should be reviewed thoroughly for laboratory results, diagnostic procedure findings, and impressions.

3. Normal reference values are established by each laboratory and should be used when evaluating the patient's test results.

4. Venous blood, and occasionally arterial collection is obtained by:
    a. Venipuncture
    b. Arterial puncture
    c. Central venous catheter blood withdrawal
    d. Capillary puncture

5. Hematological tests that are diagnostic for anemias, bleeding or coagulation problems, hemolytic disorders, or nutritional disordes include:
    a. Complete blood count (CBC)
    b. Red blood cell count (RBC)
    c. Hemoglobin (Hb)
    d. Hematocrit (Hct)
    e. White blood count (WBC)

    f. White blood differential
    g. Platelet count

6. Blood chemistry studies that are valuable indicators of homeostatic mechanisms that regulate cellular activity include:
    a. Electrolytes
    b. Blood glucose
    c. Chemistry profiles

7. Common blood coagulation studies include:
    a. Platelet count
    b. Clotting time
    c. Platelet aggregation
    d. Partial thromboplastin times (Ptt)
    e. Prothrombin time (PT)

8. Common serum enzyme assay can be used to diagnose cellular damage. Common serum enzyme studies include:
    a. Creatine kinase (heart, muscle, brain)
    b. Lactic dehydrogenase (lung, liver, kidney, heart)
    c. Aspartate amino transferase (liver, heart, skeletal muscle, kidney, brain)
    d. Alkaline phosphatase (liver, bone)
    e. Amylase (pancreas, salivary glands)
    f. Serum aminotranferase (liver)

9. Urine tests are valuable for confirming alterations in metabolism, infections, and fluid volume problems. They include:
    a. Routine urinalysis (UA)
    b. Clean catch urinalysis
    c. 24-hour urine collection

10. Culture and sensitivity testing includes:
    a. Blood cultures
    b. Urine cultures
    c. Sputum cultures
    d. Area swab cultures

F. Diagnostic tests

1. Non-invasive viewing techniques are used to visualize organs within the body and for detecting structural abnormalities. They include:
    a. Radiography
    b. X-rays using contrast media
       • Arteriogram

- Arthrogram
- Barium enema
- Barium swallow
- Bronchogram
- Cerebral angiogram
- Cholecystogram
- Intravenous pyelogram (IVP)
- Myelogram
- Upper gastrointestinal series (UGI)

   c. Fluoroscopy
   d. Mammography
   e. Radioisotope scanning
   f. Computed tomography (CT)
   g. Ultrasonography (ultrasound)
   h. Magnetic resonance imaging (MRI)

2. Invasive viewing techniques that are used to directly access a body organ or cavity include:
   a. Endoscopy
      - arthroscopy
      - bronchoscopy
      - colonoscopy
      - cystoscopy
      - fetoscopy
      - laparoscopy
      - sigmoidoscopy

   b. Angiography
   c. Cardiac catheterization

3. Aspiration procedures to obtain specimens for examination or to withdraw fluid from a body cavity include:
   a. Biopsy
      - liver biopsy
      - renal biopsy
      - bone marrow biopsy

   b. Lumbar puncture
   c. Thoracentesis
   d. Paracentesis

4. Electrical conduction studies that evaluate electrical impulses regulating body organ functions (skeletal muscle, heart, brain) include:
   a. Electrocardiography (ECG)
   b. Electroencephalography (EEG)

Unit 6

ADMISSION, DISCHARGE, AND HOME CARE

T*he patient's hospitalization is only one part of his or her health care experience. Understanding this will help guide nursing action in such a manner that a person's admission, care, and discharge can be seen as a continuous process. Hospital policies regarding admission, orientation, and discharge involve legal identification, record keeping, patient rights, and safety. At all times the individuality of the person should be maintained. This unit addresses nursing actions taken to assist patients during admission to a hospital and identifies issues of planning which are necessary for discharge and home care.*

SECTION 1: Caring for the Patient Upon Admission/Discharge and Home Care

A. Patient expectations regarding hospital admission

1. Patients expect professional competency from the health care team.
2. Most patients hope for acceptance and understanding from their care providers.
3. Patient's find themselves in a dependent position when hospitalized.

B. Patient anxiety regarding hospital admission

1. All patients will experience some degree of anxiety in response to the unknown.
2. Patient anxiety can also be generated by:
   a. The perceived position of dependency
   b. A perceived loss of control over critical decision-making ability
   c. Fear of pain and discomfort
   d. The unfamiliar and potentially threatening environment of the health care setting

C. Orientation of the patient to the institution

1. Introduce staff members as they enter the patient's room.
2. Inform the patient of the name of the head nurse or charge nurse.
3. Explain the institution's visiting hour policies.
4. Explain the institution's smoking policy.
5. Explain mealtimes, nourishment, and diet planning.
6. Explain and demonstrate all of the equipment that the patient will use.
7. Instruct the patient in the use of the nurse call light; place it in a convenient position for the patient, and have the patient demonstrate the use of the light.
8. Orient the patient to the bathroom.

D. The admission process

1. The patient's needs for care and his or her physiological condition will determine the extent to which admission procedures can be tolerated.

2. Personnel in the admitting area generally have primary responsibility for admitting patients to the institution.

3. Establishing correct, legal identification of the patient includes:
   a. Full legal name
   b. Date of birth
   c. Address
   d. Next of kin
   e. Name of the admitting physician
   f. Occupation
   g. Type of insurance or financial resources

4. The patient is assigned a permanent identifying number and issued an identification bracelet to ensure identification for all therapeutic interventions while in the institution.

5. The patient or legal guardian is advised of the patient's legal rights.
   a. A consent for treatment is obtained.
   b. Written information regarding state law involving decision-making about medical care is provided.
   c. Information about the patient's right to formulate advance directives such as living wills is discussed.
   d. Information regarding general hospital procedures and policies regarding visiting hours, pastoral services, social services, smoking policies, and other rules effecting patient conduct, is presented.

6. The patient is then transported to the nursing division.

7. The role of the nurse admitting the patient includes:
   a. Room preparation
      • Preparing the patient's room with necessary equipment and personal care items
      • Positioning the bed to safely receive the patient
      • Checking all equipment to be used by the patient for proper functioning and safety
   b. Greeting the patient and family and escorting them to the assigned room
   c. Introducing the patient to roommates, if present, nursing staff and other unit personnel
   d. Assessing the patient's general appearance, presence of signs or symptoms, and psychological status
   e. Checking the physician's admitting orders
   f. Assessing the patient's vital signs
   g. Assisting the patient to undress and get into a comfortable position

      h. Obtaining a nursing history
      i. Conducting a physical assessment
      j. Instructing the patient regarding diagnostic procedures, treatments, or other procedures scheduled for the immediate future
      k. Collecting patient valuables for safekeeping
      l. Notifying the physician of the patient's admission
      m. Providing an opportunity for the patient and family to ask questions about hospital policies, procedures, or therapies

  8. Reporting a patient's transfer within the institution.
      a. The nurse provides a review of the patient's current status.
      b. The nurse reviews all current nursing diagnoses.
      c. The nurse reviews and answers questions about the current nursing care plan.
      d. The nurse reviews and clarifies the patient's medication and treatment orders.
      e. The nurse acquires any special equipment for patient care.

E. The discharge process

  1. Planning.
      a. Discharge planning must begin when the decision is made to admit the patient to the institution.
      b. The nurse should assess the patient's acceptance of health problems and any existing restrictions.
      c. The discharge plan is based upon the patient's assessed health care needs, and the ongoing assessment of physical capabilities and cognitive functioning.
      d. The discharge plan must deal with any environmental factors within the home of the patient that might interfere with the patient's ability to meet his or her needs.
      e. Any referrals for required services must be arranged in a timely manner prior to discharge.

  2. Preparation for discharge.
      a. Patient teaching is essential for successful post institutional care, recovery, and rehabilitation.
      b. Patient teaching begins as soon as possible after admission
      c. Patient teaching issues in preparation for discharge may include:
         • Signs and symptoms of disease, illness, injury

- Signs and symptoms of actual or potential complications
- Information regarding medication therapy
- Instruction in the use of medical equipment
- Information regarding follow-up care
- Discussion of possible restrictions imposed by illness or surgical interventions

d. Make suggestions to accommodate for anticipated physical changes necessary to meet patient needs and provide a safe home environment.
e. Identify community resources available to the patient, the family, or care giver.
f. Transportation arrangements should be discussed, and made, well in advance of the actual discharge.
g. Discharge planning is focused toward:
- The patient's understanding of health problems, possible restrictions, or complications that may be experienced
- Developing the patient's ability to care for his or her needs
- Providing a safe home environment
- Identifying and activating appropriate community resources

3. Actual discharge.
a. Provide the patient, family members, or other designated caretaker, the opportunity to ask questions or discuss issues related to home care needs.
b. Review the physician's orders for prescriptions, treatments, or special equipment.
c. Assist the patient to dress for discharge and to collect all personal belongings and valuables.
d. Review previous discharge instructions with the patient and family.
e. Check that financial issues have been settled with the agency's business office.
f. Transport the patient, via wheelchair, to the institution's entrance, where external transportation should be waiting to receive the patient.
g. Make certain that patients leaving the hospital via ambulance are transported to the entrance via stretcher.
h. Document discharge and status of health problems at the time of discharge, on the discharge summary form.
i. Notify the appropriate agency departments of the time of the patient's discharge.

4. Risk factors to consider during discharge planning.
   a. The patient's or family's lack of knowledge of the treatment plan
   b. The discharge of patients with newly diagnoses chronic disease
   c. A prolonged recuperation period following illness, disease, injury, or surgical intervention
   d. The patient who is socially isolated or has limited support resources
   e. Patients who are experiencing emotional or mental instability
   f. A complex home care therapeutic treatment plan
   g. Limitations in financial resources or other access referral services
   h. The patient with a terminal illness
5. Nursing role and responsibilities in the delivery of home health care.
   a. The idea of a continuum of care has increased the importance of home care as an aspect of health care and health care delivery.
   b. If a continuum of care perspective is used as a focus for patient management, then all health team members must be aware of the patient's prioritized needs.
   c. Fragmentation of care may result in repetitious, unrelated, or inappropriate use of services, which is unacceptable.
   d. Nurses providing nursing care in the home setting provide individualized care for clients and families.
   e. Home care nursing is a very autonomous practice requiring a highly skilled individual with strong clinical decision-making skills and sound clinical judgment.
   f. Home health nurses must take the responsibility for initiating assessment, planning, implementation, and evaluation of outcomes.
   g. Effective home health nursing requires:
      • A repertoire of safe, efficient, nursing skills
      • Advanced clinical assessment skills
      • Counseling skills
      • Clinical judgment and problem-solving skills
      • Individual and group teaching skills
      • The ability to coordinate care to meet client needs and to collaborate with other health care personnel
      • A broad knowledge of community resources

- An understanding of cultural and socioeconomic factors that may influence the client's ability to meet and adhere to the treatment regimen
- An understanding of family dynamics
- Knowledge regarding home health agency regulations and policies

h. Several legal issues surround home health care nursing, including:
- Risk factors associated with the performance of highly technical procedures
- Legal aspects of client teaching involving errors and possible misuse of information provided by the nurse to the patient
- Compliance with health care provider regulations

6. Specialty home health nursing care areas.
   a. Home health care provides an opportunity for independent clinical nursing practice, teaching, and specialization.
   b. Current specialty nursing areas in home care include:
   - Hospice care
   - Home intravenous therapy
   - Respiratory home care
   - Wound care management

Unit 7

BASIC SKILLS NECESSARY FOR COMPETENT NURSING PRACTICE

The role of the nurse is to assist in the meeting of patient needs, guiding and supporting the patient, teaching, and providing an environment that fosters patient development. To accomplish this, nurses require a broad knowledge base from which to provide expert care in the face of complex and often multifaceted problems. There is a body of fundamental nursing knowledge and a set of basic fundamental nursing skills that underpin all nursing actions. Once this knowledge is established, it can then be integrated into expanded nursing activities to provide safe, competent, and effective patient care. This core of basic principles, concepts, and techniques provides the basis for the study of more advanced aspects of nursing care. The basic skills presented in this unit include: maintaining patient safety, maintaining medical and surgical asepsis, maintaining proper body alignment, promoting proper body mechanics, and the administration of medications.

SECTION 1: Maintaining Patient Safety

A. Factors that increase threats to patient safety

1. Inability to meet basic human needs.
   a. Factors reducing the amount of available oxygen include:
      - Improperly functioning heating/air conditioning equipment
      - Exposure to carbon monoxide
      - Physiological dysfunction
   b. Extremes in environmental humidity
   c. Prolonged exposure to extreme environmental temperatures, hot or cold
   d. Air pollution, water pollution, and noise pollution
   e. Physical hazards in the home
   f. Exposure to pathogens, parasites, insects, or vectors
   g. Sensory modality impairment
   h. Impaired mobility
2. Developmental age.
   a. Children under the age of five are at greatest risk for home accidents resulting in death.
   b. School age children are exposed to an expanding environment which increases the need for safety education.
   c. Adolescents are at high risk for physical accidents, alcohol and substance abuse, and suicidal behavior.
   d. Adult threats to safety are usually associated with life style choices.
   e. Among the elderly, injuries from automobile accidents, burns, and falls are the leading causes of death.
3. Life style habits contributing to unsafe conditions.
   a. Alcohol and substance abuse
   b. Smoking
   c. High stress life styles
   d. Operating machinery while under the influence of chemical substances
   e. Engaging in high risk activities
   f. Failure to follow safety instructions and precautions
   g. Failure to attend to signs of potential danger because of preoccupation with stressful concerns
   h. Lack of knowledge regarding safety
4. High-risk factors leading to falls in health care agencies involve:
   a. Neurological disorders

- Head injuries
- Spinal cord injuries
- Multiple sclerosis
- Cerebrovascular accidents
- Seizure disorders
- Brain tumors
- Parkinson's disease

b. Gait and locomotion difficulties
c. Debilitation
  - Bowel procedure preparations
  - Post-operative status
  - Invasive procedures
  - Restrictive pain
  - Diminished caloric intake
  - Prolonged bedrest

d. Mental status deterioration
  - Confusion
  - Disorientation
  - Depression
  - Organic brain syndrome

e. Central nervous system alterations
f. Sensory modality deficits
  - Blindness, use of eye patches
  - Deafness or hearing loss
  - Hemiplegia
  - Paraplegia
  - Quadriplegia
  - Proprioceptive loss

g. Debilitating diseases and disorders
  - Anemia
  - Pulmonary disease
  - Coronary artery disease
  - Cushing's disease
  - Diabetes mellitus
  - Cancer

B. Institutional environment safety

1. The patient has the right to a safe environment during hospitalization and care.

2. Because of its complexity, the health care setting is potentially dangerous.

3. Monitoring the setting for unsafe conditions and needed maintenance poses problems and requires vigilance and the assistance of the entire staff.

4. The great variety of equipment used within the facility adds to the difficulty in maintaining safety, so the nurse must be skilled in:
   a. Operating all equipment used by his or her patient
   b. Maintaining all equipment that he or she uses
   c. Detecting and correcting any problems that arise with the equipment

5. The nurse should be knowledgeable and prepared in all aspects of safety, especially the dangers of fire and natural disasters.

C. Safety within the institution

1. Many habits of safe behavior are little more than common sense.

2. Safe behaviors include:
   a. Use of good body mechanics
   b. Walking; avoiding running
   c. Keeping to the right in hallways
   d. Turning corners carefully
   e. Opening doors slowly
   f. When pushing a patient on a stretcher, keeping their head toward your body and their feet in front
   g. Using the brakes on beds, wheelchairs, and stretchers
   h. Placing elevators on "hold" when loading or unloading patients or equipment

D. Safety in working spaces, halls, and corridors

1. Areas should always be lighted at a level that ensures clear visibility.

2. Floor surfaces should be smooth and not highly polished.

3. Dropped objects should be retrieved immediately, and spills should be wiped up immediately.

4. Electrical cords should be secured in such a way that patients and staff cannot trip over them.

5. A cord or plug that is frayed should never be used because of the potential fire danger.

6. Needles and other sharp objects should be properly and promptly disposed of to prevent injuries.

7. All dangerous or caustic substances and material should be clearly labeled and properly stored.

8. Entrance doors, bathrooms, closets and cabinet doors should be fully open or fully closed to prevent people from running into them.

9. Oxygen is a gas that supports rapid combustion and should be handled with special precautions when in use in the patient's environment.

E. Protecting the dependent patient

1. Nurses should take all measures necessary to protect the dependent patient and protect him or her from injury.

2. When a bed is occupied it should remain in the low position unless a raised bed is needed for care procedures.

3. Side rails should be used thoughtfully to reduce the risk of the patient's falling out of bed.

4. Restraints should be used to protect the patient and should be used appropriately.

5. Unconscious or immobile patients must be positioned so that extremities are not caught beneath heavier portions of the body or pinned between the side rails.

6. Dropped instruments, utensils, food, nail clippings, etc. can irritate or cut the patient, and should be removed.

7. The eyes of comatose patients should be regularly inspected for, and protected from, irritation and the presence of foreign bodies; they may harm tissues or cause ulceration.

8. The patient's airway must be protected at all times to eliminate the risk of aspiration.

F. Prevention of falls within the health care agency

1. Keep the call light within easy reach of the patient.

2. Instruct the patient in the use of the emergency call bell in the bathroom.

3. Keep the patient's bedside table and over-bed table close to the patient.

4. Patients should rise slowly from the bed or chair to prevent dizziness.

5. The room and bathroom should be free of clutter and liquid spills.

6. Grab bars should be located in bathrooms, and the patient should be instructed in their use.

7. Bath mats and nonskid strips should be applied to bathtubs and shower floors.

8. Brakes on wheelchairs, stretchers, and beds should be locked while transferring patients from one to the other.

9. Canes, walkers, or crutches used by patients should be within easy reach unless supervision is required for their use.

G. Therapeutic use of restraints

1. Physical restrains are usually applied for the safety of the patient and occasionally for the protection of the staff.

2. A physician's order is required for the application of restraints.

3. All restraints must be applied with care to avoid tissue damage, restriction of circulation, and to ensure comfort.

4. The nurse must be prudent and skilled in the application of restraints.

5. Apply only the minimum restriction that will accomplish the purpose of the restraint.

6. Restraints are not used as punishment; and the patient should not be left with that impression.

7. Restraints are used to:
    a. Prevent patients from falling from bed, chairs, stretchers, or wheelchair
    b. Prevent the patient from removing tubes, dressings, or other therapeutic equipment in use
    c. Prevent the patient from scratching themselves
    d. Prevent contamination of a sterile field

8. Two types of knots commonly used to secure restraints are:
    a. The clove hitch knot, a loose knot allowing the patient some movement without restricting circulation in the body part restrained
    b. The square knot, most often used to secure a tie to the bed frame or back of a wheelchair because it does not slip

9. General considerations when applying restraints.
    a. Obtain a physician's order for restraining the patient.
    b. If the patient is already restrained, assess the need for continued restraint.
    c. When possible, provide for the patient's elimination needs before applying the restraint.

    d. Assess the amount of assistance needed to restrain the patient.

    e. Choose the restraint that best fits the needs of the patient.

    f. Always explain restraints to the patient, the uses and implications of being restrained.

    g. When a patient is restrained in bed, never tie a knot to the side rail.

    h. Padding should be used between the patient's skin and the restraint to prevent tissue damage and discomfort.

    i. Remove the restraints every two hours or less, so that the patient can be assessed, exercised, and repositioned.

    j. Evaluate the effectiveness of the restraint to ensure the correct amount of restriction.

10. Documentation should explicitly include the type of restraint used, the time it was applied, the reason for its application, the patient's physical and psychological response to being restrained, and continuous reassessment and evaluation.

11. Specific restraints commonly used in the health care setting include:

    a. Wrist or ankle restraints

    b. Body restraints

    c. Vest restraints

    d. Elbow or knee restraints

    e. Soft-tie restraints

    f. Mitt retraints

SECTION 2: Maintaining Asepsis and Controlling Infection

A. Basic principles of medical asepsis

1. Microorganisms move through space on air currents.

2. Microorganisms are transferred from one surface to another whenever objects touch.

3. Proper handwashing removes many of the microorganisms that would be transferred by the hands from one item to another.

4. Microorganisms are transferred by gravity when one item is held above another.

5. Microorganisms are released into the air on droplet nuclei when a person speaks or breathes.

6. Microorganisms move slowly on dry surfaces but very quickly through moisture.

B. Body defenses against infection

1. Normal microbial flora.
   a. Normal microbial flora reside on the skin's surface, deep epithelial structures, saliva, oral mucous, and in the gastrointestinal tract.
   b. The skin's flora exerts a decontaminating action inhibiting the growth of organisms on the skin.
   c. Flora in the mouth and pharynx impair the growth of invading organisms.
   d. Intestinal flora secrete antibacterial substances within the intestinal wall.

2. Body defenses.
   a. The intact multi-layered surface of the skin provides a mechanical barrier to microorganisms, and shedding of the outer layers removes organisms that adhere to the skin's outer layers.
   b. The saliva and mucous membranes of the mouth provide a mechanical barrier and act to wash away particles containing microorganisms.
   c. The cilia of the upper respiratory tract trap inhaled microbes and sweep them outward in mucus; macrophages engulf and destroy any microorganisms that reach the lung's alveoli.
   d. The flushing action of the urinary tract washes away microorganisms in the bladder and urethra.
   e. The low pitt (acidity) of the gastrointestinal tract chemically destroys microorganisms, and rapid peristalsis prevents the retention of bacterial contents.

3. Inflammation.
   a. inflammation is a protective vascular reaction that delivers fluid, blood products, and nutrients to the interstitial tissues of an injured area.
   b. The signs of inflammation and localized infection are: redness, localized warmth, swelling, pain or tenderness, and a loss of function in the affected body part.
   c. The signs of systemic inflammation and infection are: fever, leukocytosis, malaise, anorexia, nausea, vomiting and lymph node enlargement.

4. Immune response.

      a. The formation of immunoglobulins or antibodies is the basis for immunization against disease.

      b. Immunoglobulins provide resistance to infections.

C. The chain of infection

1. Infectious agents (resident or transient) are pathogens including bacteria, viruses, fungi, yeast, and protozoa.

2. Reservoirs are sources or places for the growth of invading pathogens and include the human body, animals, food, water, milk, plants, insects, and inanimate objects. An environment capable of supporting microorganism growth include appropriate nutrients, presence or absence of oxygen, water, a specific temperature range, a specific pH range, and the presence or absence of light.

3. A portal of entry/or exit provides the way for a microorganism to leave one host and enter another. When humans are the reservoir, microorganisms may exit through the skin and mucus membranes, respiratory tract, urinary tract, gastrointestinal tract, reproductive tract, and blood.

4. Means of transmission are the vehicles for the transmission of microorganisms and include direct and indirect, droplet contact, droplet nuclei, dust; contaminated items, food, and vectors.

5. A susceptible host is the carrier capable of supporting microorganisms.

D. The course of infection

1. The inflammatory response is a protective vascular and cellular reaction that attempts to neutralize pathogens and repair cells.

2. Signs of infection are either localized or systemic.

3. Localized infections are most commonly seen in areas of skin or mucus membrane breakdown. Abscesses are localized infections that develop in cavities beneath the skin. Signs of infection include:

      a. Redness and swelling

      b. An open lesion and possibly drainage

      c. Complaints of pain and tenderness around the site

      d. If a large area is involved, restricted movement

4. Systemic infections cause more generalized symptoms.

5. Generalized infections usually occur as a result of ineffective treatment of a localized infection. Patients may complain

of fatigue and malaise, fever, enlarged lymph nodes, swollen and tender to palpation, and often loss of appetite, nausea, and vomiting.

6. The typical course of infection.
   a. Incubation period – the interval between entrance of a pathogen into the body and the appearance of symptoms.
   b. Prodromal stage of illness – initial stage of illness evidenced by early signs and symptoms, when the host is capable of spreading the disease to others.
   c. Full stage of illness – Patient manifests signs and symptoms specific to the type of infection present.
   d. Convalescence – acute symptoms of infection disappear; period of recovery.

E. Patient susceptibility to infections

1. Susceptibility to infection changes throughout the life span.
2. Compromised and inadequate nutritional status reduces the patient's defenses against infection, delays wound healing, and increases a patient's susceptibility to infection.
3. Certain heredity conditions affect an individual's response to infections.
4. Disease processes can reduce the effectiveness of the immune system, placing patients at increased risk for infection.
5. The general adaptation response of the body to stress is a lower resistance to invading pathogens.
6. Medical therapy and drugs can compromise a person's immunity to infections.

F. Nosocomial infections

1. Nosocomial infections are those acquired during hospitalization or a stay in a health care facility. An iatrogenic infection is a nosocomial infection that occurs as the result of a diagnostic or therapeutic procedure.
2. Lack of hand washing, or improper handwashing technique, is the major cause of nosocomial infections.
3. The major sites of nosocomial infections include:
   a. Urinary tract
   b. Respiratory tract
   c. Bloodstream
   d. Surgical and traumatic wound sites

4. Invasive procedures, medical therapies, long hospitalizations, and contact with health care workers all increase the risk of acquiring nosocomial infections.

G. **Controlling or breaking the chain of infection**
   1. General aseptic measures are used to eliminate or control infections agents.
      a. Cleansing inhibits the growth of microorganisms.
      b. Disinfecting and sterilization act to disrupt the internal functions of microorganisms by destroying cell proteins.
      c. Dry heat, which disinfects but does not destroy all microorganisms, is no longer commonly used in health care settings.
      d. A combination of boiling water and stream under pressure destroys microorganisms.
      e. Ethylene oxide gas destroys spores and microorganisms by altering cells' metabolic processes.
      f. Chemical solutions such as chlorine, iodine, and alcohol are effective disinfectants.
   2. To control or eliminate reservoirs of infection:
      a. Eliminate sources of body fluids, drainage, or solutions that might contain pathogens.
      b. Use soap and water when bathing patients.
      c. Change soiled dressings or bandages, and properly dispose of them.
      d. Keep bedside units clean and dry, free of standing water, and remove open bottles of solution.
      e. Carefully assess surgical wounds and wound drainage.
      f. Use care with equipment such as suction bottles and drainage systems.
   3. To control portals of entry and exit:
      a. Carefully handle exudate such as urine, feces and emesis, wearing gloves whenever appropriate to handle these materials.
      b. Take measures to control droplet nuclei spread through sneezing, coughing, or talking.
      c. Dispose of soiled linens in proper receptacles.
      d. Maintain the integrity of skin and mucus membranes.
      e. Patients' personal items should never be shared with other patients.
      f. Linen should not be shaken or waved in the air.
      g. Wounds should be cleansed outward from the wound site.

    h. Use proper handwashing techniques.

    i. Maintain sterile technique when performing invasive procedures.

4. To protect susceptible hosts:
   a. Maintain an adequate nutritional status.
   b. Maintain adequate periods of rest, promoting sleep and comfort.
   c. Support specialized defenses, such as the cough reflex, and the normal mechanisms for urinary excretion.
   d. Educate the patient regarding infection risks, and maintain a current immunization status.
   e. Provide regular body and oral hygiene.

5. Controlling the environment.
   a. Isolation procedures include aseptic techniques and environmental barriers (masks, gloves, gowns, caps, shoe coverings, and private rooms) to confine pathogens and control infections.
   b. Patients with impaired immunity may be placed in isolation as a protective measure to prevent their exposure to microorganisms
   c. Various types of category-specific isolation procedures meet specific control purposes. These procedures stipulate the type of room and environment; gowning, gloving, masking, and other precautions to be taken by patients, personnel, and visitors.
   d. The types of category-specific isolation include:
      • Strict isolation
      • Contact isolation
      • Respiratory isolation
      • Enteric precautions
      • Acid-fast bacillus isolation
      • Drainage and secretion precautions
      • Universal blood and body fluid precautions
      • Reverse (protective) isolation.
   e. The patient placed in isolation is subject to sensory deprivation, disruption in normal interpersonal relationships, disruption in self-concept, and reduction in privacy.

H. Roles of the infection control nurse

1. Educates staff, patients, and their families on infection control

2. Reviews infection control policies and procedures

3. Screens patient's laboratory reports for culture results

4. Screens patient records for incidence of community-acquired infections

5. Gathers statistics regarding epidemiology of nosocomial infections

6. Notifies the public health department of incidence of infections and communicable disease

7. Consults with employee health departments

8. Checks results of sensitivity tests that measure the resistance of microorganism to antibiotics in use.

I. Principles of surgical asepsis

1. Areas of the body normally considered sterile are:
    a. The blood stream
    b. Spinal fluid
    c. Peritoneal cavity
    d. Urinary tract
    e. Muscles
    f. Bones
    g. Chambers of the eyes

2. Sterile objects remain sterile only when touched by another sterile object.

3. Sterile objects or fields which fall out of the range of vision or below one's waist are considered contaminated.

4. Sterile objects or fields become contaminated when they come in contact with microorganisms transported through the air.

5. Sterile objects or fields become contaminated when a sterile surface comes in contact with a wet, contaminated surface (capillary action).

6. Fluid flows in the direction of gravity.

7. Edges of a sterile field or container are considered contaminated.

J. Patient teaching issues

1. Factors increasing patient susceptibility to infections

2. The chain of infection with an emphasis on transmission of microorganisms

3. The basics of proper handwashing

4. Hygiene practices to reduce microorganism growth and spread

5. Preventive health care practices to reduce susceptibility to infections
6. Factors placing family members at risk for acquiring infections

K. Center for Disease Control Universal Precautions

1. These precautions are taken to protect health care workers from exposure to blood-borne pathogens.
2. The precautions apply to the handling of blood and other body fluids such as semen, vaginal secretions, pericardial fluid, synovial fluid, peritoneal fluid, and amniotic fluid.
3. The precautions do not apply to the handling of feces, nasal secretions, sputum, sweat, tears, urine, or vomitus unless they contain blood.
4. Barrier guidelines:
    a. Gloves should be worn when there is actual or potential contact with body fluids that may contain human immunodeficiency virus (HIV).
    b. Gloves should be removed after patient contact.
    c. Gloves should be worn when cleaning equipment.
    d. Hands should be washed between patient contacts, after any exposure to body fluids, and after removing gloves.
    e. Protective eye wear, face shields, and/or masks should be worn when there is the possibility of the presence of aerosolized blood.
    f. Gowns should be worn in emergency rooms, labor and delivery areas, surgical suites, or other areas where there is the potential for exposure to large quantities of blood.
5. Needle precautions:
    a. Never recap needles after use.
    b. Needles should never be cut, broken, or bent after use.
    c. Place used needles in appropriately labeled, impermeable needle containers.

SECTION 3: Body Mechanics, Alignment, and Mobility

A. Basic principles of body mechanics

1. When the center of gravity is maintained directly above the base of support, weight is balanced and stability can be maintained with the least amount of effort.

2. Enlarging the base of support increases the stability of the body.

3. A person or an object is more stable when the center of gravity is close to the base of support.

4. Enlarging the base of support in the direction of the force to be applied increases the amount of effort that can be applied.

5. Forming an "internal girdle", by tightening the abdominal muscles upward and the gluteal muscles downward, decreases the chance of experiencing a muscle or ligament strain or injury when lifting.

6. Turning the entire body on a plane in the direction of the task to be performed reduces spinal torsion.

7. Objects can be moved more easily on a flat surface than on a surface that is slanted or inclined against the pull of gravity.

8. Lifting is easier and less tiring when the larger leg muscles rather than smaller back muscles are used.

9. Friction between an object and the surface on which it rests should be minimized to facilitate motion.

10. Less energy is expended when holding an object close to the body than at a distance; in this way an object is also easier to move.

11. The body's weight should be used to assist in lifting and moving objects.

12. Moderate speed using smooth, rhythmical movements, requires less energy than rapid, jerky, uncoordinated movements.

13. When an object is *pushed*, soft objects (like body parts) absorb part of the force being exerted, thereby reducing the force applied and increasing the energy expended. However, when an object is *pulled*, all the force exerted is employed in moving the object.

B. Normal mobility

1. Nursing activities such as lifting, transferring, positioning, ambulating, bending standing, lying, sitting, and performing activities of daily living all require an understanding of proper body mechanics.

2. Body mechanics is the coordinated effort of the musculoskeletal and nervous systems to perform critical

functions. It is related to body alignment, balance, and coordinated movement when moving, lifting, and bending.

3. Understanding proper body mechanics requires knowledge regarding:
    a. The regulation of movement
    b. Co-ordination of body movement involving the skeletal system, skeletal muscles, and nervous system function

4. The musculoskeletal system and nervous system function to maintain proper body alignment, posture, balance, and coordinated movement.

5. Body alignment and mobility are influenced by developmental stages.

C. Assessing mobility

1. Assessing mobility provides an opportunity to determine the patient's coordination and balance while walking and performing daily activities, and can indicate his or her ability to participate in an exercise program.

2. Assessment of mobility has three components:
    a. Range of motion in joints
    b. Gait used to ambulate
    c. Exercise performance and tolerance

D. Body alignment

1. Assessment of the patient's body alignment can be performed with the patient sitting, lying, or standing.

2. The four objectives to the assessment of body alignment are:
    a. Determining normal physiological change associated with growth and development
    b. Identifying alignment difficulties associated with poor posture
    c. Assessing patient knowledge regarding posture, identifying knowledge deficits, and determining learning needs
    d. Identifying the presence of factors affecting alignment.

3. Proper alignment when standing:
    a. The head is erect and midline.
    b. The shoulders and hips are straight and parallel.
    c. The vertebral column is straight.
    d. When observed laterally, the spine curves forming a reversed "S".

    e. The abdomen is tucked in and the knees and ankles are slightly flexed.

    f. The arms hang comfortably at the person's sides.

    g. The feet are slightly apart to form a wide base of support, with the toes pointed forward.

    h. The center of gravity is midline from the middle of the forehead to a midpoint between the feet.

4. Proper alignment when sitting in a chair, wheelchair, or rehabilitation chair.

    a. The head is erect, and the neck and vertebral column are straight.

    b. Body weight is evenly distributed on the buttocks and thighs.

    c. The feet are supported on the floor or a footstool.

    d. There is a 2 to 4 cm space between the edge of the chair and the popliteal space on the posterior surface of the knee.

    e. The forearms are supported on the armrests, in the lap, or on a table in front of the chair.

    f. Avoid using pillows at the back since they might interfere with proper alignment

5. Proper alignment when lying.

    a. The vertebrae are in straight alignment, without curves.

    b. The joints are slightly flexed and supported.

    c. There should be support at the feet to prevent plantar flexion, commonly referred to as footdrop.

    d. Supports are provided along the thigh and ankles to prevent external hip rotation.

    e. A low pillow is placed under the head to prevent neck extension.

6. Proper alignment for the side-lying position.

    a. Support the head with a small pillow.

    b. Undertuck a pillow along the back to support the back and hold the patient in position.

    c. Bring the underlying arm forward, flex it, and rest it on a pillow in front of the body.

    d. The top leg should be flexed and brought slightly forward for balance.

    e. Support feet to prevent plantar flexion.

7. When positioning patients in any position, a handroll should be placed in the patient's hand with the fingers and thumb flexed around the handrail, keeping the hands in a functional position.

8. Many patients can automatically position themselves; however, they might not position themselves in a manner that promotes proper body alignment.

E. Alterations in alignment and mobility

1. Damage to any part of the musculoskeletal system or nervous system increases the risk to body alignment: joint mobility may become impaired as well.
2. A variety of factors influence body alignment and mobility.
    a. Congenital and acquired postural abnormalities affecting efficiency of the musculoskeletal system, as well as affecting alignment, balance, and appearance.
    b. Mechanisms affecting bone formation:
        • Modeling
        • Remodeling
        • Repairing
    c. Alterations in joint mobility resulting from inflammation, degeneration, or articular disruption
    d. Impaired muscle development affecting body alignment, balance and mobility
    e. Central nervous system damage affecting the regulation of voluntary movement
    f. Musculoskeletal system trauma resulting in bruises, contusions, sprains, and fractures

F. General goals for patients with alteration in body alignment

1. Maintaining proper body alignment.
2. Restoring proper body alignment, or optimal degree, of body alignment.
3. Reducing injuries resulting from impaired alignment.
4. Decreasing muscle strain.
5. Preventing deformities or complication of the musculoskeletal system or altered skin integrity.
6. Preventing contractures and foot drop.

G. General goals for patients with altered mobility

1. Maintaining full range of motion in all joints.
2. Preventing contractures in extremities, head, and neck.
3. Maintaining the patient's ability to perform daily activities.

H. Moving and positioning patients: Nursing guidelines

1. Position the bed at a height that reduces back strain.
2. Move the patient closer to one side of the bed.
3. Assess the amount of assistance necessary to safely move the patient.
4. Encourage the patient to assist in moving and positioning to their greatest potential.
5. Use aids in moving patients:
   a. Pull sheets or turn sheets
   b. Overhead trapeze
   c. Slings
6. Use large muscle groups.
7. When moving patients with the assistance of others, coordinate your movements and effort.
8. When providing patient care or performing treatments, position the patient close to the side of the bed on which you are working.
9. Use proper body mechanics when moving beds and other heavy equipment.

SECTION 4: General Principles of Medication Administration

A. Principles of medication administration

1. Appropriate precautionary measures will help avoid errors and accidents in the preparation and the administration of therapeutic agents.
2. Physiologic activities of the body can be maintained, improved, or restored by the administration of appropriate therapeutic agents.
3. A physician's order is required before administering any therapeutic agent.
4. A complete, properly written, medication order has seven essential components:
   a. Patient's full name
   b. Date the order is written
   c. Name of the medication, generic or trade name, correctly spelled

        d. Dosage, amount, or strength of the medication to be administered.

        e. Route of administration

        f. Time and frequency of administration

        g. Signature of the physician, or signature of the nurse if the order is accepted over the telephone

5. Most medication errors occur when the nurse fails to follow routine procedures.

B. Legal and ethical considerations in administering medication

1. Federal and state laws govern the use and sale of medications, and the Food and Drug Administration (FDA) enforces drug standards.

2. State's Nurse Practice Acts detail the regulations regarding nurses' roles in medication therapy.

3. Policies of health care agencies vary, and the nurse must know of the expectations regarding medication administration in his or her agency.

4. Nurses are independently licensed and take full responsibility for their actions when administering medications.

5. Drugs classified as over-the-counter medications are those that may be purchased without a physician's prescription.

6. Drugs classified as prescription medications require a physician's prescription and include medications that:

        a. May be habit-forming

        b. May produce harmful effects

        c. Require administration under the supervision of a health care practitioner

        d. Have the potential for abuse and misuse

7. Controlled substances (e.g. narcotics and barbiturates) are drugs with high potential for abuse and are closely regulated by state and federal laws.

8. It is both illegal and unethical to dispense medications without the proper license.

9. Nurses must not obtain medications for their own use, illegal use, or for the illegal use of others.

10. It is the nurse's ethical responsibility to be certain that informed consent has been obtained from the patient or their guardian when experimental drugs are administered.

C. Role of the nurse, physician, pharmacist

1. The Nurse.

   a. The nurse has primary responsibility in ensuring that medications are administratered safely and that the patient understands the medications.

   b. The nurse is responsible for building and maintaining current medication knowledge comprised of:
   - The generic and proprietary names for medications
   - Drug classifications
   - Normal drug dosages or dosage ranges
   - Appropriate route(s) for administering medications
   - Desired actions of medications
   - Common side effects of medications
   - Toxic and undesired effects of medications
   - Contraindications in the use of a medication
   - Drug incompatibilities with other medications
   - Nursing implications of the administration of medications

   c. An important responsibility of the nurse administrating medications is adherence to the "five rights":
   - Right drug
   - Right dosage
   - Right route
   - Right time
   - Right person

   d. Accurate documentation is a major responsibility of medication administration.

   e. The nurse is responsible for the appropriate safeguarding, storing, and care of medications.

   f. The nurse should always question an incorrect, incomplete, or unclear medication order, and refuse to accept an order that is considered unsafe.

   g. The nurse monitors the reordering of controlled substances.

   h. The nurse is responsible for several issues regarding the implementation of medication therapy which include:
   - Ongoing assessment that provides patient data used in diagnosis and the need for continuing medication
   - The safe administration of each dose of medication administered
   - Monitoring patient responses to medications
   - Reporting relevant patient responses, both therapeutic and negative, to health team members

2. The Physician.

        a. When ordering medications the responsibilities of the physician include:
- Taking a medical history and performing a physical examination
- Diagnosing a disease or illness requiring therapeutic intervention
- Prescribing medications to cure the disease or mitigate the disease symptoms
- Modifying medication orders

        b. The physician shares responsibility for educating patients and care givers regarding medication therapy.

        c. The physician serves as a resource of knowledge of medication therapy for members of the health team.

3. The Pharmacist.

        a. Pharmacists are highly knowledgeable in the areas of drug chemistry, classification, action, and administration.

        b. Their responsibilities in a health care agency involve selecting, obtaining, storing, and accounting for drugs, and for their safe dispensing.

        c. The role of the pharmacist is to:
- Maintain systems required for the safe administration of medications, of monitoring, documentation, and adherence to the legal requirements of medications therapy.
- Stock the pharmacy
- Check for outdated medications and solutions
- Work with nurses and physicians to educate patients

D. Rights and responsibilities of patient receiving medications

1. Patient independence and self-care should be promoted and encouraged in medication therapy.

2. Patient rights regarding the consumption of medications include:

        a. Having a complete assessment before the administration of medications

        b. Receiving complete information regarding the medications prescribed

        c. Receiving clearly identified and labeled medications

        d. Receiving notification and giving informed consent when experimental medications are prescribed

        e. Not having unnecessary medications prescribed

3. Patient responsibilities regarding medication therapy include:

        a. Understanding the therapy and questioning what they do not understand

      b. Understanding the actions necessary to adhere to the medication therapy

      c. Adhering to the therapy regimen

      d. Reporting adverse effects to medications, or change in condition

      e. Not abusing or misusing medications

      f. Properly and safely storing medications in the home

4. The nurse, acting as patient advocate, should inform the patient of their medication therapy rights and responsibilities.

E. Classification in medication therapy

1. Drugs are substances which modify or change the organism's function with or without therapeutic benefits.

2. Medications are substances that are always administered for their therapeutic benefits.

3. Oral medications are the most common type of medications administrated.

      a. Oral medications are taken by mouth for absorption in the stomach or intestines.

      b. Sublingual medications are placed under the tongue for absorption into blood vessels.

      c. Buccal medications are held inside the mouth against the mucus membranes.

4. Topical medications are applied to the skin or mucus membranes for adsorption or for local therapy.

      a. Optic medication (eye drops or ointments)

      b. Otic medication (ear drops)

      c. Nasal medication (drops or sprays)

      d. Vaginal medications

      e. Rectal medications

      f. Inhalants

      g. Transdermal medications

      h. Lotions and creams

      i. Irrigation solutions

5. Parenteral medication are given by injection with a needle. They are rapidly absorbed because of their administration directly into, or close to, either the circulatory system or site of action:

      a. Subcutaneous route – injected into subcutaneous tissues

      b. Intradermal route – injected under the epidermis into the dermis

    c. Intramuscular route – administered into muscle
    d. Intra-arterial – administered into an artery
    e. Intracardiac route – administered into the heart muscle
    f. Introsseous route – administered into the bone
    g. Intrathecal route – administered into the spinal canal
    h. Epidural route – administered into the external space of the dura mater of the spinal cord

6. Descriptions of medication effects.
    a. Therapeutic effects (desired effects) are the desired outcomes.
    b. Adverse effects or side effects of normal medication are those that are unintended or harmful.
    c. Toxic effects are adverse reactions of an overdose or abnormal accumulation of a drug in the body.
    d. Local effects are reactions affecting an area where medication has been administered.
    e. Systemic effects occur in a body organ of system distant from the site of administration.
    f. Synergistic effects are the combined effects of multiple medications given simultaneously to enhance the effects of all medications.
    g. Antagonistic effects are mutually opposing or contrary actions of two medications.

7. Various medication delivery systems have been developed for dispensing medications in the health care agency.
    a. Stock-supply system
    b. Individual cubical system
    c. Unit dose system
    d. Self medication drawers and lockers

8. Type of physician orders:
    a. Standing orders – carried out as specified until canceled by another order
    b. Single dose orders – carried out only once
    c. STAT orders – single directives to be carried out immediately
    d. PRN orders – directives to be carried out as necessary, usually at the nurse's discretion, within established parameters

F. Drug action

1. Pharmacokinetics describes the process of a medication's movement through the body, with the final stage being excretion.

2. Pharmacodynamics describes the medication's physiologic and biochemical effects on the body.
3. Pharmacokinetics involves:
   a. Absorption – process by which medication enters the blood stream
   b. Distribution – delivery of the medication to target cells and tissues
   c. Metabolism – process by which the medication is deactivated
   d. Excretion – process that removes metabolic by-products of the medication from the body.
4. Factors that influence medication action include:
   a. Patient age
   b. Patient weight
   c. Patient height
   d. Patient gender
   e. Genetic factors
   f. Time of medication administration
   g. Organ system function
   h. Patient's psychological state

G. The computing and timing of medication dosages

1. The timing of medication administration is an important aspect of medication therapy and involves:
   a. The number of doses to be given over a 24 hour period
   b. The total medication dose for a 24 hour period
   c. Pharmacokinetics
   d. Possible medication interactions with other medications, foods, or fluids
   e. Scheduling of laboratory tests or diagnostic procedures
   f. Individual needs
   g. The therapeutic goal
2. Medication orders can be written in:
   a. Volume or liquid measure
      • Apothecary system
      • Metric system
      • Household system
   b. Weight or dry measure
      • Apothecary system
      • Metric system

H. Safety measures for medication administration

1. Accurate transcription and communication of medication orders is essential.

2. When measuring liquid medication, use standard measuring receptacles.

3. When calculating dosages and conversions, avoid interferences and distractions to minimize mistakes.

4. Steps to reduce medication errors include:
   a. Read all medication labels carefully.
   b. Question the administration of multiple tables or vials for a single dose.
   c. Take caution when giving medications with similar names.
   d. Use a notification system when patients with similar names are on the same unit/floor.
   e. Double-check decimal points in dosages.
   f. Question abrupt of excessive increases, or reductions in medication dosages.
   g. When an unfamiliar drug is ordered, consult a resource for review prior to administering the medication.
   h. Do not try to decipher illegible writing in medication orders.

5. Correct administration of medications involves:
   a. Use of aseptic technique
   b. Proper adherence to regulations and procedures when administering medications
   c. Promoting patient comfort during, and following, medication administration
   d. Awareness of the need for additional measures while administering, or after administering, medication

6. The nurse never documents the administering of a medication until after it is actually administered.

7. When medications are refused by the patient, or a dose is missed, the nurse must record the reason the medication was not given.

8. Never administer a medication dose that you have not personally prepared for administration.

SECTION 5: Nursing Leadership and Management

A. Definitions of leadership and management

1. Leadership is the art of influencing people to do what the leader thinks should be done.

2. Leadership is necessary for getting a group of people to work together to accomplish a common goal.

3. Management is the art of controlling situations or environments.

4. Leaders are usually associated with:
   a. Vision
   b. Influence
   c. Innovation
   d. Social transformation
   e. Change

5. Managers are usually associated with:
   a. Improving productivity
   b. Establishing order and stability
   c. Making things run smoothly

B. Leadership and management styles

1. Leadership styles can be learned and developed.

2. There is no "best" leadership style, and no leadership style is effective in all situations. An effective leader adapts his or her style to accommodate particular situations.

3. The Authoritarian leader:
   a. Retains all power
   b. Is primarily task oriented
   c. Assigns tasks to others
   d. Establishes one-way communication patterns among group members
   e. Is characterized as being dominating, firm, insistent, and self-assured
   f. Displays little trust or confidence in others
   g. Stifles creativity and initiative of others

4. The Democratic leader:
   a. Is people-centered
   b. Delegates authority but retains responsibility
   c. Facilitates open communication
   d. Demonstrates trust and confidence in others

       e. Encourages group member participation in goal setting, decision making, and problem solving.

  5. The laissez-faire leader:
     a. Adopts a permissive leadership style
     b. Denies responsibility and gives up authority to the group
     c. Uses open, but directionless, communication channels.
     d. Abdicates goal setting, decision making, planning, and problem solving to the group

  6. The Situational leader:
     a. Directs actions of others through specific instructions
     b. Supervises task accomplishment
     c. Explains decisions, and supports progress
     d. Shares responsibility with others in the group
     e. Fosters creativity and initiative in others

C. Characteristics of an effective leader

  1. Nurses need to develop leadership and management skills early in their professional life in order to contribute to the success of professional groups, the development of health care policy, and the ensurance of quality care in a practice setting.

  2. Personal behavior skills of the effective leader.
     a. Developing a sensitivity to others' feelings
     b. Identifying with the group
     c. Being receptive to suggestions and ideas of others
     d. Fostering self-esteem and confidence in others
     e. Refraining from arguing

  3. Communication skills of the effective leader:
     a. Being an attentive listener
     b. Clarifying communication and allowing others to ask questions
     c. Establishing open, positive communication channels within the group
     d. Recognizing contributions of others

  4. Organizational skills of the effective leader.
     a. Helping the group to develop realistic goals
     b. Dividing large problems into smaller, manageable segments
     c. Sharing responsibility, authority, and opportunities
     d. Attending to details

  5. Engaging in self-examination.
     a. Reflecting on his or her own motivation

b. Developing a sensitivity to the group's culture
c. Helping group members reflect on their attitudes and values

Unit 8

CARING FOR PATIENTS REQUIRING SURGICAL INTERVENTION

In the current health care delivery setting, no area of patient care is changing quite as rapidly as that of perioperative nursing. This has occurred as the result of advancing surgical technology, less invasive surgical procedures, and a shift in the medical community's philosophy regarding the care and management of both the pre-surgical and post-surgical patient. Financial issues also play a role in this shift in persepctive. Surgery itself however, still remains a traumatic experience for the patient. Even in the face of a rapidly changing system, there continues to be a set of fundamental nursing skills required for perioperative nursing assessment, care, support, and patient education. This unit addresses the scope of practice and activities of the nurse who cares for and supports the patient at various stages of the perioperative experience. Nursing management issues involving wound care are also addressed.

SECTION 1: Providing Perioperative Care

A. Classification of surgeries

1. Surgeries can be classified according to the seriousness of the surgery, urgency of the procedure, or its purpose.

2. Seriousness.
   a. Major surgery involves extensive alterations or reconstruction in body parts and may pose great risk to the patient's well-being.
   b. Minor surgery involves minimal alterations in body parts and the physical risks to the patient are less than those associated with major surgery.

3. Urgency.
   a. Elective surgery is performed on the basis of choice; it may or may not be performed to maintain health.
   b. Urgent surgery is performed to maintain health and may be required to prevent additional health problems.
   c. Emergency surgery is done immediately to save the patient's life, maintain functioning of a body part or system, or save a body part.

4. Purpose of the surgery.
   a. Diagnostic surgical exploration allows the physician to confirm a diagnosis and may involve removal of tissue for further testing.
   b. Palliative surgery is designed to reduce the extent or intensity of a disease symptom but is not intended to cure the patient's major problem.
   c. Reconstructive surgery is performed to restore function or appearance to traumatized or malfunctioning tissues or systems.
   d. Transplant surgery is performed to replace malfunctioning organs or structures.
   e. Constructive surgery is performed to restore lost function or tissues.
   f. Ablative surgery is done to remove diseased organs.

5. Surgery may be performed in the hospital, as day surgery, in an out-patient setting, or in the physician's office.

6. The current trend is toward more day surgery, reducing the in-hospital period; this increases the educational and home care needs of the surgical patient.

B. Pre-operative surgical care

1. Preoperative preparation is an individualized process with these goals:
   a. Promoting understanding, in both patient and family, of the physical and psychological responses to surgery
   b. Promoting the return to normal function during the postoperative phase
   c. Maintaining normal fluid and electrolyte balance
   d. Minimizing contamination by microorganisms
   e. Preventing bowel and bladder incontinence during surgery
   f. Promoting rest and comfort
   g. Protecting the patient from physical harm

2. The nurse's role in the pre-operative surgical phase.
   a. Assessing the patient's physical and emotional well-being
   b. Assessing and determining the degree of surgical risks to the patient
   c. Coordinating the performance of diagnostic testing
   d. Identifying nursing diagnoses reflecting the patient's and family members' needs
   e. Preparing the patient physically, emotionally, and mentally for the surgery and the post-surgical period
   f. Communicating pertinent assessment findings to members of the health care team

3. The pre-operative nursing assessment of the patient should include:
   a. Nursing history pertaining to the surgical patient's needs
   b. Medical history focusing on past illnesses and reason for seeking care
   c. Previous surgeries and experience as a surgical patient
   d. Patient's and family members' expectations, perceptions, and understanding of the surgery
   e. The patient's medication history
   f. Identification of allergies to medications that might be used during surgery
   g. Patient's smoking pattern
   h. Patient's alcohol ingestion pattern
   i. Determination of the degree of family, friend, and social service supports available or required
   j. Occupational history
   k. Mental and emotional status examination
   l. Self-concept
   m. Coping strategies

    n. Body image
    o. Physical examination
    p. Identification of conditions and factors increasing the patient's surgical risk

4. Personal factors increasing risk for the surgical patient.
    a. Age
    b. Nutritional status
    c. Effects of radiotherapy on tissues
    d. Alterations in fluid and electrolyte balance
    e. Alteration in liver functioning
    f. Alteration in renal functioning
    g. Alteration in blood count, hemoglobin concentration, hematocrit, and volume
    h. Limitation in mobility

5. Medical conditions increasing risk for the surgical patient.
    a. Bleeding disorders
    b. Diabetes mellitus
    c. Cardiovascular disease
    d. Upper respiratory infections
    e. Chronic respiratory disease
    f. Liver disease
    g. Fever

6. Medications taken by the preoperative patient posing additional nursing implications.
    a. Antiarrhythmics
    b. Antibotics
    c. Anticoagulants
    d. Anticonvulsants
    e. Antihypertensives
    f. Antipsychotics
    g. Antidepressants
    h. Corticosteroids
    i. Insulin
    j. Diuretics

7. Informed consent.
    a. Surgery cannot be performed unless the patient understands the need for a surgical procedure, the risks involved, including risks expected as results of surgery, and alternative forms of treatment.
    b. Primary responsibility for obtaining informed consent belongs to the physician.

    c. Informed consent cannot be obtained if the patient is confused, unconscious, mentally incompetent, or under the influence of mind altering substances.

    d. Informed consent must be obtained before pre-operative medications are administered.

    e. The patient's signature on the consent form must be witnessed by another member of the health team.

    f. A consent form must be signed by the patient if:
- The patient is of legal age
- The patient is under legal age but possesses a valid marriage certificate
- The patient is designated as an emancipated minor
- The patient is not under legal guardianship

    g. If the patient is unable to sign the consent form, then properly informed parents, spouses, or legal guardians may sign.

    h. A patient has the right to refuse surgery at any time, even if informed consent has been given.

8. Structured, preoperative patient teaching should include:
    a. Ventilatory function
    b. Physical, functional capacity
    c. Sense of well-being and anxiety-reduction strategies
    d. Length of hospitalization and rehabilitation
    e. Detailed discussion, demonstration, and return demonstration of post-operative exercises or procedures
    f. Post-operative pain experience, expectations regarding pain, and proposed pain management.

9. Care on the day of surgery.
    a. Medical records are checked and charting completed.
    b. Vital signs are monitored.
    c. Hair and cosmetics are checked.
    d. Prosthetics are removed.
    e. Bowel and bladder preparations are completed.
    f. Antiembolic stocking are applied if they have been ordered.
    g. Special preparation procedures are completed:
- Specific preparation of the surgical site
- Administration of medications
- Administrative I.V. infusions
- Insertion of nasogastric or stomach decompression tubes
- Insertion of a Foley catheter

    h. Safeguarding of patient's valuables

C. Intra-operative surgical care

1. Most surgical patients will be transported to a holding area for monitoring.

2. Once admitted to the surgical area, the patient's informed consent, assessment, and medical records will be reviewed.

3. The patient will be exposed to either general or local anesthesia during this phase.

4. The patient will be positioned in a manner prescribed by the surgical procedure.

5. Positioning of the patient during surgical procedures should:
   a. Provide optimum access to the operative site
   b. Sustain adequate circulatory and respiratory functioning
   c. Not impair neuromuscular structure or functioning
   d. As nearly as possible maintain proper body alignment
   e. Permit adequate monitoring of the patient

6. Nurses in the operating room assume one of two roles with separate functions and responsibilities:
   a. The scrub nurse assists at the operative site and maintains the immediate operative area.
   b. The circulating nurse moves about the operating suite, meeting the surgical team's needs and managing unanticipated problems and needs.

D. Post-operative surgical care

1. Postoperative care is complex and requires thorough knowledge of the patient's preoperative status, type of surgical procedure performed, events occurring intraoperatively, and the anticipated recovery trajectory.

2. The postoperative course consists of two phases:
   a. Immediate recovery
   b. Postoperative convalescence

3. During the immediate recovery phase, care involves stabilizing the patient's systems most likely affected by anesthesia, immobilization, and surgical trauma.
   a. Respiration status
   b. Cardiovascular status
   c. Temperature control
   d. Restoring neurological functions
   e. Monitoring the status of surgical wounds
   f. Monitoring genitourinary function
   g. Continuing to maintain fluid and electrolyte balance
   h. Providing comfort, pain control, and rest.

4. The patient will be discharged from the recovery room and moved into the postoperative convalescence area when:
   a. Vital signs are stable
   b. Body temperature is maintained
   c. Ventilator is functioning adequately
   d. The patient is oriented to the surroundings
   e. There are no surgical or anesthetic complications
   f. There is minimal pain, nausea, or vomiting
   g. There is adequate urinary output (30ml/min.)

5. Nursing care in the postoperative phase involves:
   a. Preventing post-surgical complications
   b. Maintaining respiratory function and gas exchange
   c. Preventing circulatory stasis
   d. Promoting normal bladder and bowel elimination
   e. Maintaining adequate nutrition to promote healing
   f. Promoting rest and comfort
   g. Promoting the self-concept and, if necessary, modifying body image
   h. Promoting a return to a functional health state

E. Common postoperative complication

1. The nurse should be alert for post operative complications in all patients who have experienced surgical intervention.

2. Common respiratory system complications:
   a. Atelectasis
   b. Pneumonia
   c. Hypoxia
   d. Pulmonary embolism
   e. Impaired gas exchange

3. Common circulatory system complications:
   a. Hemorrhage
   b. Hypovolemic shock
   c. Thrombophlebitis
   d. Thrombus and embolus

4. Common gastrointestinal system complications:
   a. Abdominal distention
   b. Constipation
   c. Nausea and vomiting
   d. Ileus

5. Common genitourinary system complications
   (e.g., Urinary retention)

6. Common integumentary complications:
    a. Wound infection
    b. Wound dehiscence
    c. Wound evisceration
    d. Fistulas

SECTION 2: Principles of Wound Care

A. Wound classification

1. Wounds can be classified in terms of:
    a. Skin integrity.
        *   Open wounds with a break in skin or mucus membranes
        *   Closed wounds with no break in integrity

    b. The nature of the cause of the wound
        *   Intentional wounds resulting from therapy
        *   Unintentional, unexpected wounds

    c. The severity of the injury
        *   Superficial wounds involving only the epidermal layer of the skin
        *   Penetrating wounds involving a break in the epidermal, dermis, and deeper tissues organs
        *   Perforating wounds involving foreign objects entering and exiting an internal organ

    d. Tissue loss or no tissue loss
    e. Cleanliness
        *   Clean with no pathogens
        *   Clean contaminated, made under aseptic condition into a cavity which usually contain microorganisms
        *   Contaminated, where there is the likelihood of microorganisms present
        *   Infected with bacterial organisms in the wound site

    f. Description of the wound
        *   Laceration or tearing of tissues resulting in irregular edges
        *   Abrasion or superficial wound involving the scraping or rubbing of the skin's surface
        *   Contusion or a blow cause by a blunt object resulting in bruising, swelling, discoloration, and pain

2. Classifying wounds helps in the asssessment of risks and in nursing implications.

a. Open wounds associated with threats to skin integrity expose the patient to invasion by microorganisms, loss of blood and body fluids, and reduced functioning of a body part.

b. Closed wounds may result in internal hemorrhage, reduced functioning of an affected body part.

c. Intentional wounds made under aseptic conditions minimize the risks of infection and aid in healing.

d. Unintentional, usually traumatic wounds, occur under septic conditions, increasing the risk for infection and making healing difficult.

e. Superficial wounds increase the risk for infection, but do not involve tissue or organ injury, and usually do not affect blood supply.

f. Penetrating wounds involve a high risk for infection: They may cause internal and external hemorrhage, and the damage to underlying organs may cause temporary or permanent loss of function.

g. Perforating wounds pose a high risk for infection: they may compromise oxygenation; they may also involve serious hemorrhaging or the contamination of surrounding tissues.

h. Clean wounds pose low risk for infection.

i. Contaminated wounds pose a greater risk for infection than clean wounds.

j. Contaminated wounds usually involve tissues that are not healthy, are inflamed, and carry a high risk of infection.

k. Infected wounds present with signs of infection:
   • Inflammation
   • Purulent drainage
   • Skin separation

l. Lacerations are usually caused by contaminated objects, and complications associated with lacerations are relative to the depth of the wound.

m. Abrasions are painful and carry a risk for infection.

n. Contusions are more severe if internal organs are involved; there may be temporary loss of functioning, and localized bleeding into tissues may occur.

B. Normal wound healing

1. Wound healing involves integrated physiological processes.

2. All wounds heal in the same manner with some difference depending on location, severity, and extent of the injury.

3. Wound healing is affected by tissue growth and regeneration.

4. Wounds heal by either primary intention, secondary intention, or tertiary intention.
   a. Primary intention involves healing of areas with little or no tissue loss, close approximation of wound edges, and low risk for infection.
   b. Secondary intention involves healing of areas of tissue loss, wound edges that do not approximate, areas left open until filled with scar tissue, prolonged healing, and chances for infections are high.
   c. Tertiary intention occurs when wounds close after the wound surface has started to granulate; the result is deeper and wider scar formation.
5. Wound healing occurs in three stages:
   a. The defensive stage begins immediately and usually lasts 4 - 6 days; reparative processes work to control bleeding, deliver blood, and form epithelial cells at the injury site.
   b. The reconstructive stage involves wound closure with new tissue and can last 2-3 weeks.
   c, The maturation stage, which can last up to a year, is the final stage of healing when collagen fibers undergo remodeling and organization.

C. Complications when wounds fail to heal properly

1. Hemorrhage.
   a. Hemorrhage can occur internally or externally.
   b. Hemorrhage after initial homeostasis has occurred can be an indication of a slipped suture, dislodged blood clots, infection, or erosion of a blood vessel.
   c. External hemorrhaging is identified by observing dressings for bloody drainage.
   d. Internal hemorrhaging can be detected by observing for distention or swelling of the affected area or for signs of hypovolemic shock.
2. Dehiscence.
   a. Dehiscence is a partial or total separation of the layers of the wound and should be considered a medical emergency.
   b. Dehiscence is a sign of improper wound healing.
   c. Obese patients and patients with abdominal incisions are at greatest risk for wound dehiscence.
   d. An increase in serosanguineous drainage can be an indicator of wound dehiscence.

3. Evisceration.
   a. Evisceration is the protrusion of visceral organs through the wound opening and is considered a medical emergency requiring surgical intervention.
   b. Protrusion through the wound opening compromises the organ.
   c. Sterile towels soaked in sterile saline should be draped over the protruding tissues to decrease microorganism invasion and tissue drying.
4. Fistulas.
   a. A fistula is an abnormal passage between two organs or between an organ and the outside of the body.
   b. Fistulas can be created surgically for therapeutic purposes, but most are the result of a failure in wound healing, trauma, infection, or disease.
   c. Fistulas can result in infection, electrolyte and fluid imbalance, and skin breakdown.
5. Infection.
   a. Infection is present if purulent material drains from the wound.
   b. Wound infections are the most common types of nosocomial infection.
   c. The chances for infection are greater:
      • When the wound contains dead or necrotic tissue
      • When foreign bodies have entered the wound or are near the wound
      • When blood supply and tissue defenses are lowered
   d. Bacterial infection hinders wound healing.
   e. Signs of wound infections include:
      • Fever
      • Tenderness and pain at the wound site
      • Elevated white blood cell count
      • Inflamed wound edges
      • Purulent drainage
      • Wound culture containing microorganisms

D. Factors influencing wound healing include:

1. Age
2. Nutrition status
3. Obesity
4. Extent of the wound
5. Oxygenation

    6. Smoking behavior

    7. Immunosuppression

    8. Diabetes

    9. Wound stress

    10. Drug intake

E. Nursing assessment

The nursing assessment of wound sites should focus on:

1. Normal skin status
2. Risks for impairment of skin integrity
3. Identification of altered skin integrity
4. Inspection of the wound includes
   a. General appearance, size, shape
   b. Classification of the wound
   c. Drainage system device, open or closed system, patency
   d. Wound drainage, type, amount, color, consistency, and odor
   e. Patient complaints of tenderness, pain, or a sense of "pulling"
5. Signs associated with the various complications associated with wound healing

F. Objectives and management of wound care

1. Principles of skin care.
   a. Skin must be adequately hydrated.
   b. The body's cells require adequate nourishment.
   c. The body's cells require adequate circulation.
   d. Hygiene is essential to maintaining skin integrity.
   e. Health status is an important factor in skin sensitivity.
2. Objectives of wound care include:
   a. Promoting wound homeostasis
   b. Preventing infection of the wound site
   c. Preventing further injury to the wound
   d. Supporting wound healing
   e. Maintaining skin integrity
   f. Promoting normal functioning
3. Dressings, protective coverings thatabsorb drainage, prevent contamination and mechanical injury, maintain pressure and immobilize the wound. They include:
   a. Permeable dressings

    b. Semipermeable dressings or composite dressings

    c. Occlusive dressings

    d. Transparent dressings

    f. Hydrocolloids

    g. Hydrogels and gels

    h. Calcium alginate dressings

4. Mechanisms for supporting wound areas and preventing stress and tension on the incision include:

    a. Sutures and staples

    b. Clips

    c. Bandages

    d. Steristrips and butterflies

    e. Binders

5. Maintaining effective drainage systems provide a track to eliminate drainage from wounds and reduce the risk for complications, they include:

    a. Ensuring patency of drains

    b. Recharging drains

    c. Advancing drains

6. Other wound care products that the nurse should be familiar with include:

    a. Nonionic cleansers

    b. Exudate absorbers

    c. Skin barriers

    d. Wound deodorizers

    e. Enzymatic debriding agents

    f. Stimulating sprays

    g. Leg ulcer wraps

7. The nurse should know various types of dressings, types of wound products, and wound support mechanisms, in order to ensure that appropriate measures are selected to facilitate wound healing.

8. Wounds healing by secondary intention may require:

    a. Debridement – the physical removal of foreign material or dead tissue from a wound

    b. Irrigation – the flushing of a wound with a solution to clean out exudate or debris

    c. Packing – the insertion of sterile packing to prevent the wound from closing prematurely, reducing the risks of infection and abscess formation

9. The "Ostomy" nurse has advanced training and knowledge regarding the care of wounds and skin care. The Ostomy

nurse either provides direct wound care for patients or serves as a consultant for nurses responsible for skin and wound care.

G. Principles of hot and cold application

1. Physiological responses and the therapeutic uses of heat.
   a. Blood vessels in the wound area dilate causing increased blood circulation, enriched oxygenation to the tissues, and improved tissue metabolism.
   b. Heat can be used to:
      - Relieve pain from muscle spasms and affected joints
      - Reduce swelling by increasing circulation
      - Eliminate toxic waste products that accumulate in the area of swelling or edema
      - Relax muscles
      - Promote healing by increasing oxygenation and promoting suppuration in the presence of infection

2. Physiological responses and the therapeutic uses of cold.
   a. Cold causes blood vessels to constrict.
   b. This constriction slows circulation which may:
      - Reduce hemorrhage or oozing
      - Decrease pain through its anesthetic effect on skin
      - Reduce inflammation when applied locally
      - Prevent the formation of edema

3. Safety issues related to the application of heat and cold.
   a. Patients vary in their tolerance to heat and cold.
   b. Length of exposure time to heat or cold, as well as size of the skin area involved, affects tolerance to the application of both heat and cold.
   c. Skin temperature receptors adjust rapidly to even mild stimulation.
   d. Increased pain and swelling, decreased sensation, mottling, or extreme redness may be indicators that the application should be stopped.
   e. When applying heat, affected areas should be checked at least every 20 minutes.
   f. Air is a poor conductor; moisture conducts heat better than air.

H. Methods for applying heat and cold therapy

1. Dry heat.
   a. Water-flow heating pads with control units or aquathermia pads
   b. Electric heating pads

      c. Hot water bottles
      d. Disposable hot packs
      e. Heat cradle
      f. Heat lamp or infrared lamp
      g. Diathermy

2. Moist heat.
      a. Warm compresses or wet dressings
      b. Soaks or immersion of a body part
      c. Sitz baths to soak the perineal and rectal areas
      d. Paraffin baths
      e. Hydrocollator packs

3. Cold.
      a. Ice collar or ice cap
      b. Cold compresses
      c. Disposable cold packs
      d. Cooling sponge bath
      e. Hypothermia blanket

Unit 9

SPECIAL PATIENT PROBLEMS AND NURSING MANAGEMENT ISSUES

R*egardless of the area of nursing specialty, there is a group of common patient problems which the nurse can expect to encounter in clinical practice. Often nursing plays a pivotal role in preventing and managing these patient problems. Pain is a significant universal experience encountered in every field of nursing. It is a subjective phenomenon often misunderstood by the nurse and, as research would support, an area that is often ineffectively managed by nurses. Illness, injury, disease, and hospitalization all create conditions which foster extreme distress and anxiety, dangers from immobility, and disruptive, cognitive disorganization. If properly managed, patients who experience these problems will not be subjected to additional complications from health care services or hospitalization.*

SECTION 1: Management of the Patient Experiencing Pain

A. Nature of pain

1. Nurses frequently care for patients experiencing pain.
2. Pain can interfere with every aspect of living, working, playing, eating, sleeping, thinking, etc.
3. Perception and interpretation of pain stimuli occur at the cortical level of the brain.
4. The threshold at which individuals experience pain varies widely, and personal reactions and responses to pain differ greatly.
5. The threshold for pain is often high in people with apathetic or stoic temperaments, low in high-strung, nervous individuals.
6. Pain is a subjective intrapersonal experience.
7. Pain is a protective physiological mechanism, a warning that something is wrong.
8. While pain is a common problem encountered by nurses in practice, it is often a frustrating experience for both the nurse and the patient.

B. Pain perception

1. The pain experience is a three stage process:
   a. Reception – the neurophysiological component
   b. Perception – the awareness of pain sensation and its interpretation
   c. Reaction – the physiological and behavioral response
2. The physiological responses to pain involve sympathetic and parasympathetic nervous system stimulation.
3. The signs and symptoms of parasympathetic stimulation (most often encountered with superficial pain) involves:
   a. Blood shifting away from the periphery
   b. Muscle tension and fatigue
   c. Vagal stimulation
   d. Rapid, irregular breathing
   e. Nausea and vomiting
   f. Weakness or exhaustion
4. The signs and symptoms of sympathetic stimulation (most often experienced with deep pain) involves:

      a. Dilation of bronchial tubes and increased respiration
      b. Decreased heart rate
      c. Peripheral vasoconstriction
      d. Alteration in blood glucose level
      e. Pupil dilation
      f. Decreased gastric motility

5. Sources of physical pain include:
      a. Trauma
      b. Ischemia
      c. Irritation
      d. Alteration in body fluids
      e. Duct distention
      f. Perforation of a visceral organ
      g. Space-occupying lesions
      h. Burns

6. The nurse's goal in the management of pain is to control or intervene at any one of the three stages of the pain process.

7. Patient behavioral responses to pain include:
      a. Crying
      b. Moaning
      c. Sighing
      d. Yelling and swearing
      e. Guarding the painful part
      f. Facial grimacing
      g. Withdrawal and isolation
      h. Rubbing or massaging the affected part
      i. Holding the affected part
      j. Rhythmic rocking

8. Types of pain experienced by patients.
      a. A classification system of pain experiences can assist in decision-making regarding pain management interventions.
      b. Superficial or cutaneous pain – resulting from stimulation of the skin that is of short duration, localized, and usually experienced as a sharp sensation.
      c. Deep visceral pain – resulting from stimulation of internal organs is diffuse and may radiate; its duration is usually longer than superficial pain, and its sensation may be sharp, dull, or unique.
      d. Referred pain – resulting from the brain's perceiving pain in an unaffected area; may assume any characteristic.

e. Radiating pain – a sensation of pain extending from the initial site of injury to another body part; it feels as though it travels down or along a body part, and may be intermittent or constant.
f. Phantom pain – is an abnormal sensation or feelings in an amputated body part; it can continue long after the incision site heals.
g. Neurogenic pain – result of peripheral or central nervous system damage, so that any sensation is perceived as pain; most often perceived as a burning sensation.
h. Psychogenic pain – originates in the mind, sources can be fantasy, wishes, needs, impulses involving ideas of injury or punishment; it can involve the mental defense mechanism of conversion. Psychogenic pain does not fit into any currently understood anatomic pattern. It recurs at precise intervals under certain conditions or under emotional stress. It is not relieved by ordinary analgesic measures. Symptoms cannot be explained by the presence of demonstrable organic disease or structural abnormalities.

C. Acute and chronic pain

1. The pain threshold is the point at which an individual first perceives the painful stimuli. It is the intensity of stimuli required for pain to be perceived or experienced.
2. Pain tolerance is the point at which an individual will react to pain with verbal or other responses.
3. Experience with acute pain.
   a. It is usually of brief duration.
   b. The onset is immediate.
   c. It has an expected end.
   d. The pain may subside with or without intervention.
   e. It is a new and often frightening experience.
   f. It typically evokes overt behavioral responses from the patient.
4. Acute pain can be a serious threat, an obstacle to a patient's recovery, and should be considered a priority patient problem.
5. Experience with chronic pain.
   a. The pain begins as an acute pain or as an increasing discomfort.
   b. The pain lasts a prolonged period of time.
   c. The pain experience is unpredictable.

    d. There can be periods of remission and exacerbation of the pain.

    e. The pain may never be completely controlled.

    f. The experience causes extreme frustration and may lead to psychological depression.

6. The experience of chronic pain can result in psychological and physical disabilities leading to:

    a. Job loss

    b. Disruption in interpersonal relationships

    c. Divorce

    d. Inability to perform activities of daily living

    e. Sexual dysfunction

    f. Social isolation

    g. Disruption in meeting personal goals

    h. Loss of self-esteem

D. Pain assessment and importance in nursing care

1. Pain is always ascribed to a body location.

2. A key to successful pain assessment is not to ignore the patient's report concerning their pain experience.

3. The pain experience is essentially subjective; however certain characteristics of pain measured objectively.

4. During an episode of acute pain, assessment is focused primarily on the patient's physiological responses, location, severity, and quality of the pain.

5. A thorough pain assessment takes time, and should be performed when the patient is comfortable and can cognitively attend to the nurse's questions regarding pain.

6. A complete assessment of the patient's subjective report of the pain experience includes location, severity, quality, time and duration, precipitating and aggravating factors, relieving factors, and past experiences with pain.

7. Identifying location is the first step in pain assessment.

    a. Identify the location of the pain.

    b. Generally superficial pain is easier to locate than visceral pain.

    c. Pain location can be characterized as being:

      • Localized

      • Diffuse

      • Referred

      • Radiating

     d. Ask the patient to point to the most severe point of the pain and trace it outward.

     e. Knowledge of underlying disease and illness can help to locate the origin of pain.

     f. Anatomical landmarks and descriptive terminology should be used when describing and documenting pain location.

8. Intensity is the most subjective characteristic of the pain experience.

     a. Pain can be subjectively described as being mild, moderate, or severe.

     b. An objective way to assess pain severity is by using a descriptive scale, ranking the pain on a scale from 0 (slight) to 10 (intense).

     c. A descriptive scale can be useful in monitoring changes in pain severity.

9. Quality is the description of the perceived stimuli.

     a. Pain can be described as being:
   - Sharp
   - Throbbing
   - Dull
   - Crushing
   - Burning
   - Stinging

     b. The nurse should use the patient's description of the pain's quality when documenting assessment data.

10. Timing and duration are assessed to determine the onset, periodicity and duration of pain, and should be measured as accurately as possible.

11. Precipitating events and aggravating factors can be helpful in planning interventions to avoid exacerbating pain. Precipitating events and aggravating factors can be disease- or illness-specific and can include:

     a. Physical exertion and exercise

     b. Emotional distress

     c. Eating

     d. Bending, stretching, lifting, twisting

     e. Work related tension

     f. Urinating

     g. Jarring or vibration

     h. Swallowing, talking

     i. Rubbing, scratching

     j. Coughing and deep breathing

    k. Environmental extremes

12. Relieving measures are helpful in planning pain management and control, and may include:
    a. Position change
    b. Application of hot or cold
    c. Eating or drinking
    d. Rest
    e. Analgesics
    f. Distraction
    g. Guided imagery
    h. Accupressure

13. A pain history should include a thorough description of past pain experiences.
    a. Determine whether episode is acute or chronic.
    b. Note recollections of the pain experience.
    c. Identify past pain relieving measures the patient used and the effectiveness of those measures.
    d. Identify the patient's meaning assigned to the pain.

E. Therapeutic intervention for control and management of pain

1. Guidelines for individualizing pain management.
    a. Attempt different types of pain relief measures.
    b. Provide pain relief measures prior to the point at which the pain becomes severe.
    c. Use pain relief measures that the patient thinks are effective.
    d. Assess the patient's willingness to actively participate in pain relief measures.
    e. Use pain relief measures that are appropriate for the patient's subjective report of the severity of the pain.
    f. Attempt a pain relief measure more than one time if it is not initially effective.
    g. Keep an open mind about pain relief measures.

2. An awareness of the influence of pain on the patient's normal functioning and life style helps in the identification of practical approaches to pain management.

3. The nurse's goal in the management of pain is to control or eliminate any one of the three components of the pain process (See part B. Pain perception, above).

4. Measures to prevent pain reception.
    a. Removing a painful stimuli from the environment is a long- lasting and extremely effective strategy.

- Remove wet, irritating dressings
- Loosen bandages
- Apply heat to increase circulation
- Change activity patterns
- Administer muscle relaxants
- Apply padding over bony areas before applying restraints or bandages.

   b. Prevent exposure of the skin to chemical stimuli and caustic substances.
- Keep the skin of incontinent patients dry.
- Apply ointments and barriers to protect skin.

   c. Prevent exposure to thermal stimuli.
   d. Lift patient up in bed rather than pulling them.
   e. Identify and avoid precipitating events and aggravating factors.
   f. Reduce the extent to which pain receptors are exposed using bandages, padding or local anesthetics.

5. Measures to lessen pain perception.
   a. Application of gate control therapy measures such as the application of cutaneous stimulation.
- Massage or backrub
- Warm bath
- Application of hot and cold
- Application of liniments

   b. Do not use cutaneous measures in cases involving burns, rashes, bruising, inflammation, and underlying bone fractures.
   c. Increase the input of meaningful sensory stimuli so that the patient focuses on stimuli other than the pain.
   d. Provide distraction.
- Music
- Hobbies and crafts
- Television

   e. Administer analgesics.
   f. Suggest hypnosis for psychogenic pain.
   g. Use biofeedback techniques.

6. Measures to modify the pain reaction.
   a. Modifying anxiety associated with pain helps to relieve pain and to potentiate the effects of other measures.
   b. Relaxation provides mental and physical relief from tension or stress and promotes a sense of self-control during the pain experience.

c. Guided imagery requires that the patient use all the senses to concentrate and create an image which reduces awareness of pain.

7. Measures to alter interpretation and response to pain
   a. Administer narcotics.
   b. Administer hypnotics.
   c. Increase interactions between the patient and nurse.

8. Medical measures can be used to provide temporary or permanent pain relief.
   a. The characteristics of an effective analgesic include:
      • Rapid onset
      • Long-term effectiveness
      • Effectiveness with all ages
      • Multiple routes of administration
      • Freedom from severe side effects
      • Nonaddictive properities
      • Affordability
   b. Using a regular schedule for analgesic administration can help prevent intense pain experiences.
   c. Local anesthetics produce a loss of sensation, motor function, and autonomic nervous response, by inhibiting nerve conduction.
   d. Placebos bring about pain relief even though there are no direct physiological or chemical effect on the patient.
   e. Surgical procedures are used to relieve persistent pain when it is clear that the source of pain is physiological. These procedures include:
      • Surgical resection of nerve pathways
      • Blocking impulse transmission
      • Acupuncture
      These medical measures are used in combination with other therapies and complement nonpharmacological nursing interventions.

8. Evaluation of pain management requires observations regarding:
   a. The changing character of pain
   b. The patient's response to interventions
   c. The patient's perceptions of the effectiveness of therapeutic interventions
   d. The level of patient functioning and sense of comfort and control

SECTION 2: Managing the Immobile Patient

A. Mobility and immobility

1. Mobility is the individual's ability to move about freely.

2. Complete mobility requires voluntary motor function, balance and coordination.

3. Partial mobility results from sensory alteration or motor dysfunction in a region of the body.

4. Partial mobility can be a temporary or permanent condition.

5. Immobility is the inability to move about freely because of a restriction in movement.

6. Four conditions can result in immobility:
   a. Physical inactivity resulting in reduction in body movement, such as bedrest
   b. Imposed reduction in movement, such as the application of a cast
   c. Alteration in body position and posture, reducing ability to adapt to such changes
   d. Sensory deprivation, such as hemiplegia

7. The degree of disruption due to immobility is relative to the duration of the immobile state.

B. Benefits and hazards of bedrest

1. Bed rest is an intervention which restricts the patient to bed for therapeutic reasons.

2. The therapeutic benefits of bed rest include:
   a. Reducing physical activity
   b. Reducing the oxygen needs of body tissues
   c. Reducing pain
   d. Providing an opportunity for ill or debilitated patients to rest and regain strength
   e. Providing uninterrupted rest, relaxation, and sleep for overworked or very stressed patients
   f. Promoting wound healing
   g. Providing proper skeletal alignment

3. The potential hazards of bed rest include:
   a. Physiological alteration
   b. Psychological and emotional alterations
   c. Safety concerns

4. Examples of conditions requiring bed rest include:
   a. Acute myocardial infarction

   b. Congestive heart failure
   c. Head injuries
   d. Spinal cord trauma
   e. Degenerative neurological conditions
   f. Muscle strains and sprains
   g. Torn ligaments
   h. Fractures
   i. Infection

C. Responses to altered mobility

   1. Every body system is at risk for alterations resulting from immobility.
   2. The severity of the impairment will depend on age, health status, duration, and severity of the immobility.
   3. The potential hazards of bedrest include:
      a. Normal metabolic equilibrium disruption
         • Decreased metabolic rate
         • Tissue atrophy and protein catabolism
         • Fluid and electrolyte changes
         • Bone demineralization
         • Alteration in gas exchange
         • Alteration in gastrointestinal functioning

      b. Respiratory alterations
         • Decreased lung expansion
         • Pooling of secretions in the lungs
         • Difficulty in deep breathing and coughing

      c. Cardiovascular alterations
         • Decreased stability and balance
         • Orthostatic hypotension
         • Increased cardiac workload
         • Thrombus and phlebitis formation

      d. Musculoskeletal alterations
         • Decreased activity endurance
         • Decreased muscle mass and tone
         • Atrophy
         • Formation of contractures
         • Osteoporosis

      e. Integument alteration
         • Formation of decubitus ulcer

      f. Elimination alteration
         • Formation of renal calculi
         • Urine stasis

- Urinary tract infection
- Kidney infection
- Decreased gastrointestinal mobility
- Constipation
- Fecal impaction

g. Psychological responses
- Irritability
- Depression
- Changes in sleep-wake cycle
- Decreased coping abilities
- Decreased problem solving abilities
- Increased isolation
- Sensory deprivation
- Decreased cognitive functioning and disorganization
- Increased dependence

D. General goals for patients with alteration in mobility

1. Goals focusing on potential metabolic alterations include:
   a. Maintaining adequate nutrient intake consistent with any imposed dietary requirements or restrictions
   - High-protein diet
   - High-caloric diet
   - Vitamin C supplement

   b. Maintaining fluid balance
   c. Preventing muscle wasting

2. Goals focusing on potential respiratory function alterations include:
   a. Maintaining an open airway
   - Deep breathing and coughing exercises
   - Nasotracheal or orotracheal suctioning if appropriate
   - Adequate hydration
   - Humidifying room air and oxygen
   - Proper patient positioning

   b. Maintaining lung expansion
   - Repositioning the patient every 2 hours
   - Deep breathing and coughing exercises

   c. Preventing stasis of pulmonary secretions
   - Repositioning patient every 2 hours
   - Chest physiotherapy

   d. Providing humidity and moisture

3. Goals focusing on potential cardiovascular alteration include:
   a. Maintaining cardiac output during postural changes

- Perform leg exercises
- Apply elastic stocking
- Dangle at bedside before getting out of bed
- Getting out of bed as soon as appropriate given the patient's physical condition
- Dangle at bedside as appropriate given the patient's physical condition

b. Reducing cardiac workload
   - Using overhead trapeze when moving and positioning
   - Scheduling procedures, tests, or therapy to provide rest periods

c. Promotion of venous return
   - Encourage proper positioning to prevent pressure on deep leg veins.
   - Incorporate routine exercises into daily activities.
   - Use elastic stockings.
   - When bathing the patient's extremities, use long firm strokes toward the center of the body.

4. Goals focusing on potential musculoskeletal alterations include:
   a. Maintaining the present level of joint range of motion
      - Perform passive or active range of motion exercises routinely.
      - Encourage the patient toward self-care and to participate in activities as appropriate, given their physical condition.

   b. Decreasing the patient's activity intolerance
      - Engage in a progressive exercise program.
      - Use devices to assist in ambulating and moving.

   c. Promoting tolerance to weight-bearing activities
      - Engage in a progressive exercise program.
      - Use devices to assist in ambulating.

5. Goals focusing on potential integument alterations include:
   a. Maintaining skin integrity
      - Assess pressure points every 1 - 2 hours.
      - Reposition the patient every two hours.
      - Maintain smooth bed linens.
      - Use mechanical devices to reduce pressure.
      - Use devices such as flotation pads, sheepskin, pillows, and trochanter rolls, to support specific pressure areas.
      - Keep the skin clean and dry.

   b. Reducing the duration of pressure

- Develop a 24-hour turning schedule.
- Use devices which minimize or equalize pressure; these include alternating air mattresses, water mattresses, Clinitron beds, egg crate mattresses

   c. Reducing the skin irritation
- Keep skin clean and dry.
- Use skin care products as appropriate.

6. Goals focusing on potential elimination alterations include:
   a. Maintaining adequate fluid intake
   b. Maintaining adequate nutritional intake
   c. Maintaining proper bowel and bladder functioning
   d. Preventing bladder distention
   e. Preventing constipation and bowel impaction

7. Goals focusing on psychological adjustment to immobility include:
   a. Promoting normal coping patterns
   b. Promoting normal sleep-wake cycle
   c. Promoting socialization
   d. Providing adequate, meaningful stimuli
   e. Encouraging diversional activities as appropriate
   f. Promoting physical, mental, intellectual stimulation appropriate to the patient's physical condition

SECTION 3: Management of the Patient Experiencing Grief and Loss

A. Normal (conventional) grief response

1. Loss is a universal experience that occurs throughout the life span.

2. A significant loss can be categorized as:
   a. Actual or perceived
   b. Objective versus subjective
   c. Material versus psychological
   d. Expected versus unexpected
   e. Maturational versus situational

3. Any change that is perceived by the patient as a negative change in the way they relate to their environment can be considered a loss of self.
   a. Loss through growth and development

      b. Self-concept challenged, with loss of physical or mental capabilities

4. In primitive societies death was accepted as a normal, natural event; however in contemporary society, death is often a hidden, isolated, unacceptable event.

5. Grief is a form of sorrow involving feelings, thoughts, and behaviors caused by bereavement.

6. Responses to loss are strongly influenced by one's cultural background.

7. When a grieving individual finds openness, encouragement, and support in others, he or she can develop understanding and personal growth.

8. The nurse's own feelings, values, and personal experience with loss can greatly influence his or her ability to assist patients experiencing loss.

9. Grief can serve several functions:
   a. Making the outer reality of the loss into an internally accepted reality
   b. Severing the emotional attachment to the lost object or person
   c. Making it possible for the bereaved individual to reorganize their lives and replace lost objects

10. Mourning involves the cultural, ethnic, spiritual rituals, and socially prescribed behaviors which help people to acknowledge loss.

11. The grief process involves a sequence of affective, cognitive, and physiological states as a person responds to, and finally accepts a loss.

12. "Grief work" refers to the mourning process and involves:
    a. Somatic distress
    b. Disengagement
    c. Reinvestment through loss resolution

13. Responses to loss and patterns of coping with loss are developed early in life.

B. Major theories of the grieving process

1. Theoretical frameworks for understanding grief can be process oriented or behavior oriented.

2. Engle's theory.
   a. This theory is a process oriented theory which incorporates three steps.

    b. The first step is denial and disbelief.
- The individual denies the reality of the loss.
- The individual may withdraw from others, sit motionless, or wander aimlessly.
- Physical reactions may include fainting, diaphoresis, nausea, diarrhea, increased heart rate, restlessness, insomnia, and fatigue.

    c. The second step is developing awareness.
- The individual begins to feel the loss acutely and may experience a sense of desperation.
- Emotions experienced may include anger, guilt, frustration, depression, and a feeling of emptiness.
- The person may become preoccupied with the loss.
- Crying is typical behavior at this step.

    d. The third step involves the acknowledgment of the loss and the reorganization of one's life without the lost object.

3. Kubler-Ross's theory.

    a. This theory is behavior oriented and incorporates three stages.

    b. During stage one, denial, the individual acts as though nothing has happened and refuses to believe that the loss has occurred.

    c. During stage two, anger, the individual resists the loss and may "act out" feelings.

    d. During stage three, bargaining, the individual attempts to make deals in an attempt to postpone the reality of the loss.

    e. During stage four, depression, the full impact of the loss is felt and there may be overwhelming feelings of loneliness and withdrawal from others.

    f. During the final stage, acceptance, the individual comes to terms with the loss, or impending loss, physiological reactions to the loss cease, and interaction with others can be resumed.

4. Glasser and Strauss's theory.

    a. This theory focuses on the trajectory of the dying process.

    b. Four trajectories are proposed:
- Certain death at a known time
- Certain death at an unknown time
- Uncertain death but with time for assessing whether there is a life threatening situation

- Uncertain death without time for assessing whether there is a life threatening situation
5. Lindemann's theory.
   a. This theory focuses on a common pattern of the grief experience.
   b. Six reactions to a loss are identified:
      - Somatic distress
      - Preoccupation with the image of the deceased
      - Guilt
      - Hostile reactions
      - Loss of patterns of conduct
      - Appearance of traits of the deceased
6. Park's theory.
   a. This theory identifies grief as a complex process that is individual, interactive, physical, emotional, and environmental.
   b. Park perceives grief as a major life transition, manifested by:
      - Numbness as an initial response to the loss
      - Intense yearning for the deceased person or lost object
      - Disorganization of daily life
      - Reorganization and restructuring of a new life pattern
7. Grieving is an individual experience and the person may not pass through every stage identified in these theories, nor might they progress through the stages in a sequential, predetermined manner.
8. Behaviors characteristic of identified stages may be anticipated, but are not to be expected of every individual responding to a loss.

C. Common misconceptions about death and dying

1. No one is willing to die, unless he or she is suicidal or psychotic.
2. No one can help another accept death since reconciliation with death and preparation for death are impossible.
3. Fear of death and dying is a fundamental fear.
4. The closer one is to death the greater the sense of fear.
5. When dying patients do not ask about their prognosis, they do not want to know about it.
6. Only the physician has the knowledge and skill to deal with terminal care.

D. Categories of loss

1. The grief process is similar across individuals regardless of the nature of the loss.

2. A major loss requires a long term adjustment period and life transition.

3. A loss can be a personal loss, a group loss, or a community loss.

4. Loss can be categorized as:
   a. Loss of external objects
   b. Loss of an aspect of the self
   c. Loss of a significant other
   d. Loss of the self through death
   e. Loss of a known environment

E. Anticipatory grief response

1. An anticipatory grief response is a pattern of behavior that a person may affect when faced with an impending loss.

2. Anticipatory grieving may aid in coping with the loss when it occurs.

3. The nurse must guard against the premature "social death" of a patient when anticipatory grieving occurs prior to physical death.

4. Nurses often can assume the role of significant others in cases where anticipatory grieving has occurred and separation from family members occurs prematurely.

F. Unresolved grief response

1. The person acts as though the loss event never occurred.

2. By denying the loss, and not grieving, the individual can refuse to acknowledge the pain associated with the loss.

3. Painful effects of the loss may be replaced by inappropriately good spirits and pleasure.

G. Factors influencing a reaction to loss

1. When assessing the grieving patient, the nurse must focus on the meaning of the loss to the patient.

2. Growth and developmental stage play a major role in responding to loss.
   a. Infants and toddlers lack the cognitive maturity to develop an understanding of loss and death. They respond most often with feelings of anxiety.

    b. The majority of pre-schoolers may perceive death as a type of sleep, or as a temporary separation.

    c. Often the school age child associates death with misdeeds, or bad thoughts, and may experience intense feelings of guilt when a death occurs. The school age child has the cognitive maturity to understand an explanation of death. The school age child also has the beginning of a body image and will experience grief over the loss of a body part or function.

    d. Adolescents experience acute grief when confronted with a loss of a body part or function. Adolescents can develop an adult understanding of death; however they are the least likely of any age group to accept death.

    e. Young adults relate loss to status, role, and life-style. Their concept of death is generally shaped by religious or cultural beliefs.

    f. Middle-aged adults become aware of their own mortality, sensing that time is at a premium and that life is finite.

    g. The elderly experience anticipatory grief resulting from physical changes of aging and the fear of a loss of independence. The elderly person's response to loss will reflect their sense of life fulfillment and worth. The elderly person requires a longer period of grief work due to a shorter time to reorganize their lives after a loss, and difficulty in replacing lost objects.

3. Factors influencing the response to a loss include:

    a. Values and feelings ascribed to the object

    b. Nature of the pre-death relationship when the lost object is a significant other

    c. The circumstances under which the loss occurred

    d. Personal resources and other stressors
- Physical and mental health status
- Coping skills
- Previous experience with loss
- Emotional stability
- Spiritual beliefs
- Family developmental stage
- Socioeconomic status

    e. Sociocultural resources and stressors
- Cultural mores and societal customs
- Available social support network
- Self-help groups
- Hospice programs
- Bereavement programs
- Pastoral counselors

H. Dysfunctional grieving

1. A dysfunctional grieving response falls outside of the normal behavioral range usually demonstrated by individuals experiencing a lose.

2. Dysfunctional grieving can be seen as:
   a. Exaggerated grief
   b. Prolonged grief
   c. Absence of grief

3. The grieving person is unable to progress through the grief process and expends a great deal of energy repressing grief or ineffectively dealing with grief.

4. Dysfunctional grief results in the disruption of everyday life activities, work, and relationships.

I. Normal and abnormal grief responses

1. Normal behavior during the first year of bereavement include:
   a. Excessive or persistent expressions of affect
   b. Inability to experience joy and happiness
   c. Clinical symptoms of depression
   d. Inability to form new relationships
   e. Expression of emotion when talking about the deceased person
   f. Perception of hearing or seeing the deceased person
   g. Expression of feelings of meaninglessness or emptiness
   h. Dreams of the lost object
   i. Identification with the lost object
   j. Seeking and pining for the lost object

2. Abnormal behavior when present beyond three years of the loss include:
   a. Preserving the deceased's room and belongings intact
   b. Reporting similar physical symptoms as those experienced by the deceased
   c. Talking about the loss as though it had occurred recently
   d. Preoccupation with thoughts of the deceased
   e. Talking about the deceased in the present tense
   f. Inability to attend to daily activities and responsibilities

3. Caution should be taken when labeling a patient as manifesting the characteristics of a dysfunctional grief response.

J. Awareness of impending loss

1. People facing loss possess varying degrees of awareness of the impending event.

2. Three degrees of awareness have been identified:
   a. Closed awareness – The patient and family appear unaware of the reality of the extreme severity of the situation. Health care providers fail to communicate diagnosis or prognosis. There can be no discussion of the impending loss.
   b. Mutual pretense – Everyone involved in the impending loss is aware of the reality of the situation but do not talk about it. No attempt is made to raise issues associated with the impending loss. There is a sense that the family is trying to protect the patient or that the patient is trying to protect the family. The results are the inability to verbalize fears and concerns and the loss of necessary supports. Mutual pretense is emotionally draining for everyone, including staff, and places a great strain on interpersonal relationships.
   c. Open awareness – Everyone is aware of the impending loss and comfortable about discussing it, even though it is difficult to confront. This type of awareness allows planning and finalizing affairs. Everyone involved can participate in solving problems, making plans and decisions. Individuals can resolve conflicts, and say their good-byes.

K. Nursing management to promote functional grieving and mourning

1. Interventions should be based on a knowledge of the long-term nature of the grieving process.

2. Nursing management is directed toward promoting the patient's sense of identity, dignity, and self-esteem.

3. General goals related to the management of the patient experiencing loss and grief include:
   a. Maintaining self-esteem
   b. Promoting a return to life activities
   c. Providing comfort and safety for the dying patient
   d. Maintaining the independence of the dying patient
   e. Conserving the dying patient's energy
   f. Promoting spiritual comfort for the dying patient and family
   g. Supporting the grieving family and mobilizing social resources

4. Physical and psychological health and adjustment during the grieving process are closely related

5. Discharge planning should include consideration of the long term nature of the grieving process.

6. The outcome of an experience with loss cannot be predetermined; it is the result of balancing the stressors present and the resources available during mourning.

7. Hospice programs are important resources providing family oriented support for those experiencing grief.
   a. The hospice views the family as the unit of care.
   b. The quality of life is more important than its quantity.
   c. The needs of the dying patient are complex and are provided by an interdisciplinary team of care providers.
   d. Interventions are focused on management of physical and psychosocial needs of the patient and the family.

L. Assessment of the patient in a state of impending death

1. Reflexes gradually disappear.

2. Cheyne-Stokes respiration pattern occurs.

3. Facial expression may be pinched.

4. Skin becomes cold and clammy.

5. Pupils becomes dilated and fixed.

6. Pulse slows and becomes increasingly weak.

7. Blood pressure drops.

M. Caring for the dying patient

1. Emotional care.
   a. Provide relief from loneliness, fear, and depression.
   b. Maintain security, self-confidence, and dignity.
   c. Maintain hope, but do not give false reassurance.

2. Spiritual care.
   a. Needs will reflect the patient's relationship with a supreme being or association with an organized religion.

3. Physiological care.
   a. Observe for signs of cyanosis.
   b. Administer analgesics I.V. rather than subcutaneous or intramuscular.
   c. Provide warmth.
   d. Administer Oxygen therapy to relieve respiratory distress.
   e. Frequently reposition the patient.

4. Care related to loss of muscle tone.
   a. Provide padding for urine and fecal incontinence.
   b. Suction accumulated mucus from the mouth and provide frequent oral care.
   c. Provide relief from nausea, vomiting, and flatus due to decreased peristalsis.
   d. Maintain body alignment.
      • Place the conscious and semi-conscious patient in a Semi-Fowler's position.
      • Place the unconscious patient in a Semi-prone position.
   e. Reduce edema formation by preventing body parts from being placed in dependent positions.
5. Care related to alteration in the sensory modalities.
   a. Monitor lighting as vision becomes blurred and finally fades.
   b. Protect the patient from pain and physical discomfort.
   c. Provide frequent eye care.
   d. Monitor noise levels; hearing appears to be the last sensory modality to cease.
   e. Talk to the patient, providing comfort and security.
   f. Provide physical contact through touch.
6. Care related to alteration in respiration.
   a. Position the patient to facilitate breathing and lung expansion.
   b. Suction as necessary.
   c. Administer oxygen as ordered to ease distress.

SECTION 4: Management of the Patient Experiencing Cognitive Disorganization

A. The nature of cognitive disorganization

1. Cognitive disorganization, usually in the form of confusion, is frequently encountered by the nurse.
2. The nurse is the first line of defense against cognitive disorganization in the health care setting.
3. Cognitive disorganization is a rapidly progressive patient state.
4. Early prophylactic interventions and early detection of cognitive impairment are essential.

5. The most common behaviors demonstrated by patients experiencing cognitive disorganization include:
   a. Confusion
   b. Disorientation
   c. Hallucinations – Perception in the absence of an external stimuli.
      Example: Hearing voices when no one is in the room.
   d. Illusions – Misinterpretation of an existing stimuli
      Example: Thinking that an I.V. pole is a person standing at the foot of the bed.
   e. Delusions – Thoughts not grounded in reality
      Example: A patient's belief that a nurse is her dead sister.

B. Confusion

1. Confusion generally refers to a state of disordered orientation, a disturbance in the sense of time, place, person.

2. Confusion can have organic or psychic causes.

3. Disorientation is the impairment of spatial, temporal, or personal relationships.

4. Disorientation to person, the inability to know one's own identity, is the most severe form of disorganized thinking.

5. The comatose patient cannot be confused or disoriented.

6. Confusion is a less severe alteration of brain function.

7. Confusion can often be a transitory experience, making it difficult to assess. A series of observations made over time is required to accurately diagnosis confusion.

8. The confused person is frightened, feels defenseless, and is afraid of being taken advantage of.

9. Restraining or forcing the confused patient will heighten their fear, confusion, defensiveness, and aggression.

10. Cognitively disorganized patients are impulsive and unpredictable.

C. Assessment issues when interviewing the confused patient

1. Verbal and non-verbal cues should be used when assessing the patient's degree of confusion.

2. Be certain that appropriate questions are asked.

3. Be certain that the patient is fully awake.

4. Be certain that the patient has access to required aids to orientation.
    a. Glasses
    b. Hearing aid
    c. Additional lighting
5. Be certain that the patient is attentive to the nurse and the interview process.
6. Be certain that the patient and interviewer speak the same language.
7. Be certain that the patient does not have physical impairment for speaking, comprehending, or memory retrieval.

D. Risk factors for cognitive dysfunction

1. Factors that increase the likelihood of impaired processes include physiological, psychological, and environmental risks.
2. Confusion can be classified as irreversible or reversible.
    a. Irreversible causes of confusion include:
       • Alzheimer's disease
       • Multi-infarct Dementia
       • Benign senescent forgetfulness
    b. Reversible causes of confusion include:
       • Physiological conditions
          1. Infection
          2. Elevation in temperature
          3. Altered thyroid function
          4. Altered glucose metabolism
          5. Calcium imbalance
          6. Hyponatremia
          7. Hypokalemia
          8. Vitamins and mineral deficits
          9. Anemia
          10. Pernicious anemia
          11. Hypoxia
          12. Cranial tumors
          13. Increased intracranial pressure
          14. Head trauma
       • Psychological conditions
          1. Depression
          2. Stress and anxiety
          3. Sensory alterations
       • Iatrogenic causes
          1. Drugs
          2. Self-fulfilling prophecies

      3. One way to organize the risk factor for potential cognitive disorganization is by the use of the phrase "MEND A MIND".

        a. Metabolic disorders
        b. Eating disorders
        c. Neurological impairment
        d. Dehydration
        e. Anemia
        f. Medication toxicity
        g. Infections
        h. Neoplasm
        i. Decreased sensory acuity

3. Sensory deprivation is the greatest risk factor for confusion among the hospitalized elderly population.
   a. They are often isolated.
   b. They experience a normal decrease in sensory modality acuity associated with aging.
   c. They often have nutritional deficits and dehydration.
   d. They are frequently taking medication that can contribute to cognitive disorganization.
   e. They often engage in self-medication behavior.

E. Common behaviors that are often associated with confusion

1. Paranoia and insecurity.

2. Accusing other of stealing from them.

3. Hoarding behavior as a means of establishing a sense of control. Objects hoarded may hold some meaning for the patient.

4. Compulsiveness as an adaptive strategy for coping with loss and diminished capabilities
   a. Excessive orderliness
   b. List-making
   c. Writing everything down

F. General goals related to care of the patient with disorganized cognitive functioning

1. Create an environment that facilitates cognitive functioning.

2. Focus on providing an environment that supports the patient in the presence of existing impairments.

3. If impairment exists protect the patient from harm.

G. Nursing measures for problems of cognitive disorganization

1. Prevention
   a. Keep the patient oriented to the environment.
      - Use clocks and calendars large enough to be easily read.
      - Remind the patient of the day and date as necessary.
   b. Provide consistency in the care-giver assignment.
      - Keep patient oriented care-givers.
      - Provide one "anchor person" to provide care for the patient.
      - Assign a person who will frequently be available to the patient and can spend periods of time with the patient.
      - The care-giver should be a non-coercive individual who will include, rather than exclude, the patient in care activities.
   c. Communicate with the patient.
      - Keep messages to the patient clear and concise.
      - Obtain feedback from the patient on messages communicated.
      - Engage in goal-directed conversation with the patient.
      - Speak in a calm voice audible enough for the patient to hear without effort.
      - Constantly inform the patient about activities in which he or she will be involved.
      - Provide explanation regarding procedures, sounds, equipment, noises, and odors in the patient's environment.
      - Always call the patient by his or her name.
      - Do not rush the patient to perform activities of daily living or communication.
      - Use touch as a means of communicating.
   d. Reduce extraneous noise, light, and other distractions.
   e. Provide a safe environment.
      - Provide adequate lighting.
      - Use restraints as appropriate.
      - Keep room and hall free of clutter.
      - Use side rails at all times.
   f. Provide the patient with his or her own belongings.
      - Pictures
      - Clothing
      - Personal hygiene items
      - Blanket (if permitted)

- Be certain as to whether the patient wears glasses, dentures, or hearing aids.
- Be certain that the hearing aids have functioning batteries and that glasses are clean.

g. Maintain a predictable routine or schedule.
h. Encourage meaningful activities and interactions with others.
i. Provide positive reinforcement for behaviors that show increased orientation.

2. Support and protect the patient with identified impairment
   a. The confused patient is not acting for the staff's benefit. NEVER laugh at the confused patient; it will confuse the patient further.
   b. The room and hallways should have adequate light.
   c. Lighting should vary for day and night.
   d. A night light should be provided.
   e. Aids to orientation should be provided.
      - Radio and television with schedule for use.
      - Newspapers and magazines
      - Eye glasses clean
      - Hearing aid turned on with functioning batteries
      - Personal clothing and hygiene items
      - Personal pictures, cards, notes, flowers
   f. Rearrange room furniture, and/or position the patient, so that he or she may observe unit activity.
   g. Provide a variety of meaningful stimuli.
   h. Decrease noise, shadows, and drafts.
   i. Closely supervise the patient.
      - Monitor hydration.
      - Monitor nutritional intake.
      - Monitor level of activity tolerance.
      - Monitor bowel and bladder function.
   j. Turn and reposition patient frequently, altering bed position.

3. Reorientation.
   a. Help to reestablish the reality that the patient shares with others.
      - Talk about real things instead of abstract concepts.
      - Talk about real facts of concern to the patient.
      - When feeding the patient talk about foods that are on the tray.
      - Stress shared time: day, date, time at each encounter with the patient.

- Repeatedly identify yourself to the patient.

b. When talking with the confused patient:
  - Get and retain their attention.
  - Speak slowly.
  - Face the patient and maintain eye contact.
  - Use the appropriate tone of voice.
  - Speak as an adult.

c. Help the patient get to sleep without medications.
  - Provide a back rub.
  - Have a brief conversation.
  - Attend to the patient's elimination needs.
  - Provide warm milk if there is no dietary restriction.

d. Discourage social isolation.
  - Provide communal dining for ambulatory patients.
  - Coordinate patient group games and activities.
  - Arrange visitations with other patients in the dayroom.
  - Encourage participation in rehabilitative activities.
  - Encourage participation in patient outings.

H. When the patient's confusion is irreversible

1. Establish a stable, structured environment.

2. Employ reality orientation and memory cues consistently.

3. Provide for safety within the environment.

4. Use the patient's name frequently.

5. Establish physical contact with the patient during communication.

6. Encourage physical involvement in activities of daily living.

7. Encourage mental activity through games, activities, and diversion.

I. Managing the agitated patient

1. Agitation is frequently encountered in the health care setting and is one of the most difficult behaviors to manage.

2. Two of the most frequently used nursing interventions for dealing with this disorganized behavior—restraints and administration of tranquilizers—may actually agitate the patient further.

3. Agitation can often be prevented by taking steps to minimize anxiety and promote a sense of control.

    4. Providing opportunities for the patient to make decisions is extremely beneficial for combating feelings of loss of control associated with agitation.

    5. Specific nursing measures for managing the agitated patient include:

        a. Remaining calm to foster reassurance

        b. Reducing stimuli to a minimum

        c. Approaching the patient calmly from the side, never from the front

        d. Identifying yourself when approaching the patient

        e. Using a calm, monotonous voice to reassure the patient that things are under control

        f. If physical contact is possible, hold the patient from the side and use a rocking motion for its calming effect on the patient

        g. If tranquilizers must be administered by injection, prepare the patient by using simple, clear language.

SECTION 5: Management of the Patient Experiencing Anxiety

A. The nature of anxiety

    1. Emotions are feelings that prompt an observable reaction to internal mental and physiological changes.

    2. Anxiety has been referred to as the motivating emotion.

    3. Anxiety is psychic energy.

    4. Anxiety is mental distress in anticipation of some future threat or danger.

        a. The source of anxiety is vague.

        b. The threat is internal.

        c. Anxiety can exist for an extended period of time.

        d. Anxiety is the consequence of psychological conflict.

    5. Fear is an emotional response to a present danger.

        a. Fear is caused by a specific, recognizable source.

        b. The source of the threat is external.

        c. Fear is concerned with the present.

        d. The source of fear is definite.

        e. Fear is not the consequence of psychological conflict.

    6. Emotions exist on three levels:

        a. Neuroendocrine

      b. Motor-visceral
      c. Conscious awareness.

7. Emotions are not observable, but their physiological and behavioral results are.
    a. Increased brain wave activity
    b. Increased heart rate
    c. Muscular tension and irritability
    d. Increased respiration
    e. Increased renal function

8. Perception beginning in infancy (7-8 months of age) is key in understanding anxiety.

9. Anxiety forces change and is the driving force in all human adjustment.

10. Anxiety is an essential part of life and can be harmful or helpful depending on:
    a. Its degree of intensity
    b. Its appropriateness in the context of a person's experience
    c. Its duration
    d. Ability of the person to cope with and reduce anxiety

B. Factors leading to anxiety

1. Anxiety is generated by anything that threatens the physical or mental security of the individual.

2. Primary causes of anxiety are:
    a. Frustration over obstacles that block goal satisfaction
    b. Conflict which arises in the presence of incompatible desires, wishes, prestige, status, or goals
    c. Threats to biological integrity.

3. Physical threats are more easily identified than threats to the self-concept.

4. Anxiety, which is highly contagious, is always transmitted through interpersonal contact.

C. Symptoms of anxiety

1. Epinephrine is released during anxiety.

2. Heart rate and depth of respiration increase.

3. Rapid shifts occur in:
    a. Blood pressure
    b. Body temperature
    c. Urinary urgency

      d. Menstrual cycle and flow

4. The patient can experience:
   a. Dry mouth
   b. Back pain
   c. Chest pain
   d. Headache
   e. Decreased appetite
   f. Nausea, vomiting, and diarrhea

5. Pupils dilate, and the liver releases sugar.

6. Libido may decrease and impotency may occur.

D. The degrees of anxiety as a continuum

1. Anxiety can be seen as ranging from the lowest level (apathy) to the highest level (panic).

2. The levels of anxiety are often ranked as described numerically from 0 (low) to +++ (high).

3. Understanding the degree of anxiety and the disruption to normal homeostasis that may exist at each level is helpful in the management of patient care.

4. Ataraxy or apathy.
   a. This is the lowest level of anxiety.
   b. It denotes the absence of anxiety.
   c. This absence of anxiety can be drug induced.
   d. The patient will not be motivated to take any action in this state.

5. Relaxation or well-being.
   a. This state generally follows satisfying experiences.
   b. The person feels relaxed, comfortable, and happy.
   c. The person is not very alert to the environment.
   d. This state is believed to be therapeutic.

6. Mild anxiety (+)
   a. This is a gentle level of anxiety.
   b. It is the level of anxiety experienced by most productive, creative, healthy individuals.
   c. At this level anxiety is an asset to successful adaptation.
   d. At this level the individual is interested and attentive.
   e. This is the best state for learning.

7. Moderate anxiety (++) or intermediate.
   a. At the lower end of this level there is a heightening of perception and increased attention to cognitive and physical abilities.

   b. At this level the individual prepares to learn.

   c. At this level the individual can also prepare to flee.

   d. As anxiety rises at this level there is a narrowing of perception, decreased awareness, and inattention to peripheral activities.

   e. The person begins to feel uneasy, nervous, or tense.

   f. The person will either be willing to confront the sources of anxiety, or try to evade them.

   g. If he or she is willing to face the anxiety during this level, intervention may have the greatest chance of success.

   h. Personal growth and behavior modification is best achieved at this level of anxiety.

8. Severe anxiety (+++).

   a. This is an intense, very painful, and harsh state.

   b. This is not a useful condition and the aim should be to reduce the feelings of anxiety.

   c. The person's creative or productive energy is consumed in trying to cope with the feeling of anxiety.

   d. This level of anxiety inhibits restoration.

   e. The person is too "keyed up" to concentrate.

   f. The person feels helpless, isolated, insecure, and disorganized.

   g. The person cannot see his or her life experience as a whole picture, rather as disconnected pieces.

9. Panic anxiety.

   a. This is a frightening state.

   b. The person has a sense of disintegration and loss of control.

   c. This is a critical condition and requires immediate intervention.

   d. The person cannot perceive accurately, make decisions, remember, control affect, or control motor activities.

   e. Communication is severely disrupted.

E. Behavior patterns used to control anxiety

1. "Acting out".

   a. Acting out is the overt use of anger to help identify the details necessary to justify anger.

   b. Acting out prevents the recognition of anxiety or the source of the anxiety.

2. Reporting psychosomatic disorders.

3. "Freezing to the spot".

   a. Responding to anxiety by withdrawal, depression.

  b. Choosing to take no action.

 4. Using anxiety's energy to enhance learning.

  a. Enduring anxiety while searching for causes of the emotion

  b. Enduring the anxiety while struggling through the problem

 5. Using defense mechanisms to defend and bolster self-esteem.

  a. Defense mechanisms are used unconsciously.

  b. They are characterized by such characteristics as self-deception, and the masking of true motives.

  c. They are used to deny drives and impulses that might cause anxiety.

  d. They are used to distort perception, memory, actions, and motivation.

  e. Defensive mechanisms are neither good nor bad in nature; they serve as protective devises for the ego.

  f. An understanding of how patients use defense mechanisms helps in understanding their fears and concerns.

F. Nursing measures for reducing patient anxiety

 1. Help the patient work through their anxiety.

  a. Develop awareness of anxiety by exploring the patient's feelings, and sensations.

  b. Help the patient confront his or her anxiety.

  c. Help the patient focus on, recognize, and name the source of anxiety.

  d. Help the patient to develop insight into the anxiety experience.

   • Explore the nature and meaning of the perceived threat to the patient's physical or psychological well-being.

   • Conduct reality testing to gauge the degree of the perceived danger.

   • Estimate the likelihood that the perceived threat will actually occur.

   • Distinguish fact from fantasy.

  e. Explore new ways for the patient to cope with anxiety.

   • Support group involvement.

   • Use direct communication.

   • Increase self-esteem.

   • Develop effective problem-solving approaches.

f. Help the patient regain a sense of control and security.
    *   Decrease ambiguity or uncertainty in the environment.
    *   Provide stability, especially for patients experiencing high levels of anxiety.

g. Manipulate the anxiety-producing environment.
    *   Lower the amount of stimuli to a tolerable level.
    *   Communicate with the patient using simple, clear, concise statements.
    *   Give the patient only essential information; do not overload them with information.
    *   Temporarily reduce decision-making demands.
    *   Provide a physically safe environment.
    *   Provide a calm, consistent care giver.

h. Provide an appropriate outlet for muscular tension.

Bibliography

Berger, K.J. and Williams M.B. (1992). *Fundamentals of Nursing Collaborating for Optimal Health.* Norwalk, Connecticut: Appleton & Lange.

Bolander, V.B. (1994). *Sorensen and Luckman's Basic Nursing A Psycholophysiologic Approach.* Philadelphia: W.B. Saunders Company.

Craven, R. F. and Constance, J. H. (1992). *Fundamentals of Nursing Human Health and Function.* Philadelphia: J.B. Lippincott Company.

Ellis, J.R. and Nowlis, E.A. (1994). *Nursing: A Human Needs Approach.* Philadelphia: J.B. Lippincott Company.

Potter, P.A. and Perry, A.G. (1993). *Fundamentals of Nursing Concepts, Process & Practice.* St. Louis: Mosby Year Book, Inc.

R

Record keeping
  purposes of, 40
Recording and reporting, 40
Reporting
  change-of-shift, 41
Respiration, 101
Restraints
  therapeutic use of, 122
Risks for surgical patient, 150
Role, 12
  ambiguity, 14
  conflict, 14
  strain, 14
  stressors, 14

S

Safety and security needs, 62
Self-actualization needs, 64
Self-concept, 10
  altered, 14
Self-esteem, 12
Self-esteem needs, 64
Self-esteem stressors, 13
Signs of altered family function, 7
Spiritual distress, 16
  signs of, 16
Spiritual health, 16
  nursing process, 17
Spiritual needs
  assessment of, 18
Spirituality, 16
Stress, 68
  psychophysiological
  response to, 71
Surgeries
  classification of, 148
Surgical asepsis, 129
Susceptibility to infections, 126
Systemic infections, 125

T

Task roles, 8
Teaching principles
  basic, 46
Teaching-learning process, 44
Telephone reporting, 42
Therapeutic communication, 36
Therapeutic nurse/patient
relationship
  phases of, 37
Topical medications, 139
Types of communication
  nonverbal, 36
  verbal, 35

U

Universal precautions, 130
Unresolved grief response, 180

V

Values, 18
  formation of, 19
  modification of, 19
Verbal communication, 35
Vital signs
  assessment of, 98

W

Wound care, 154
Wound classification, 154
Wound healing, 155

Skidmore-Roth Publishing, Inc. Order Form
1(800) 825-3150

Qty.	Title	Price	Total
	The Nurse's Trivia Calendar	$ 9.95	
	PN/VN Review Cards, 2nd ed.	$24.95	
	The Nurse's Survival Guide, 2nd ed.	$24.95	
	The Drug Comparison Handbook, 2nd ed.	$26.95	
	Oncology/Hematology Nursing Care Plans	$27.95	
	The Skidmore-Roth Outline Series: Diabetes	$16.95	
	The Skidmore-Roth Outline Series: Geriatric Nursing	$16.95	
	RN NCLEX Review Cards, 2nd ed	$24.95	
	AIDS Nursing Care Plans	$27.95	
	AIDS Instrant Instruct	$15.95	

Tax of 8.25% applies to Texas residents only. UPS ground shipping $5 for first item, $1 each additional item.	Subtotal	
	8.25% Tax	
	Shipping	
	TOTAL	

Name	
Company	
Address	
City	
State	Zip
Phone	

____ Check enclosed	____ Visa	____ MasterCard
Credit Card Number		
Card Holder Name		
Signature	Expiration Date	

For fastest service call, 1-800-825-3150 or fax your order to us at (915) 877-4424. Orders are accepted by mail. Prices subject to change without notice.

Skidmore-Roth Publishing, Inc.
7730 Trade Center Avenue
El Paso, TX 79912